# A Theory for Nursing

# A Theory for Nursing

## SYSTEMS, CONCEPTS, PROCESS

**Imogene M. King, Ed.D., R.N.**

Professor
College of Nursing
University of South Florida
Tampa, Florida

**A Wiley Medical Publication**
John Wiley & Sons
New York • Chichester • Brisbane • Toronto

Copyright © 1981 by John Wiley & Sons, Inc.

This work includes some material previously published by the same author in a book entitled: *Toward a Theory for Nursing*. Copyright © 1971, John Wiley & Sons, Inc.

All rights reserved. Published simultaneously in Canada.

Reproduction or translation of any part of this
work beyond that permitted by Sections 107 or 108
of the 1976 United States Copyright Act without the
permission of the copyright owner is unlawful. Requests
for permission or further information should be addressed
to the Permissions Department, John Wiley & Sons, Inc.

**Library of Congress Cataloging in Publication Data:**

King, Imogene M.
   A theory for nursing.

   (A Wiley medical publication)
   Includes bibliographies and index.
   1. Nursing—Philosophy.  I. Title.  II. Series: Wiley medical publication.  [DNLM: 1. Philosophy, Nursing. 2. Systems theory.  WY 86 K52t]

RT84.5.K55      610.73′01     81-1996
ISBN 0-471-07795-X         AACR2

Printed in the United States of America

10 9 8 7 6 5 4 3 2 1

To my family, colleagues, and students,
and to those nurses who will conduct
the research to test this theory
in nursing situations

# Preface

This book was written to promote conceptual learning in undergraduate and graduate nursing programs, whose students will find the book helpful in three ways. First, it presents a conceptual framework by linking concepts essential to understanding nursing as a major system within health care systems. Second, it offers one approach to developing concepts and applying knowledge in nursing. Third, it demonstrates one strategy for theory construction by presenting a theory of goal attainment derived from the conceptual framework.

The original framework, published in *Toward a Theory for Nursing,* presented several major concepts in three dynamic interacting systems that suggested interrelationships among individuals, groups, and society. The same systems framework is presented in this book, with additional concepts identified and developed as relevant content for nursing. Ideas from the first book have been used in this volume. The goal of this systems framework for nursing is helping people maintain their health. A concept of health is presented, including promoting health practices, preventing disease, caring for those who are ill and dying, and providing health teaching and guidance for people so that they can maintain their ability to function in their usual roles.

A special feature is the presentation of a goal-oriented nursing record that was constructed to demonstrate a systematic approach to documenting nursing care. This approach provides a method to preserve an accurate record that can be used to measure the effectiveness of nursing care. Several examples of nursing problems related to medical problems are identified and nursing diagnoses made. In addition, in cooperation with clients, the information gathered is used to identify goals, to determine the means to achieve them, and to record accurately the progress toward achieving the goals. This systematic and theoretical approach to the practice of nursing demonstrates both the independent functions of professional nurses and their collaborative activities with other health professionals.

An additional purpose of the conceptual framework is to facilitate the transition from the role of student to the role of nurse. This can be done because of the concepts identified and developed within social systems. Knowledge of the concepts of organization, power, authority, status, and decision making is essential if nurses are to understand formal and informal organizational structures in health care systems.

Many excellent books focus on nursing care of people with illness, disease, and disability. This book offers a necessary companion to all textbooks because it suggests a systems approach for the structure of the discipline of nursing. The concepts presented in the framework and in the theory provide a way of understanding human beings as individuals interacting with other individuals within a variety of environments and influenced by perceptions, roles, past experiences, and concrete situations.

A conceptual framework for nursing is presented in Chapter 1. Within the framework, concepts have been identified and developed as substantive knowledge for nursing in Chapters 2, 3, and 4. A theory of goal attainment derived from the conceptual framework and the descriptive phase of testing the theory are shown in Chapter 5. In Chapter 6, a goal-oriented nursing record, with suggestions for forms on which to record nursing care, is offered as one approach to documenting the effectiveness of nursing care.

It is hoped that the framework presented here will encourage readers of this book, both students and professional nurses, to test the theory further.

I.M.K.

# Acknowledgments

The conceptual framework and the theory in this book are a synthesis of many people's ideas. I want to thank students, faculty members, and colleagues who have listened to these ideas, discussed them with me, and raised questions that helped to clarify some of the abstractions.

I am grateful to the four graduate students, Lynn Antoniou, Cynthia Burns, Patricia Egel, and Diane Smith, who requested an experience in nonparticipant observations and collected the descriptive data for the initial testing phase of the theory. To all graduate students who have applied these ideas in becoming clinical specialists and have provided feedback to me, thank you.

My sincere appreciation is extended to Dr. Jacqueline Fawcett for a constructive and helpful critique of the manuscript and for being a true colleague. The kindness of Cathy Somer, former nursing editor at John Wiley & Sons, is greatly appreciated. Thanks to my nieces Donna Buckley, for providing editorial assistance, and Carol Menke, for proofreading and commenting on the manuscript.

I.M.K.

# Contents

## 1. A Conceptual Framework for Nursing   1
What Is Nursing?   2
What Is the Goal of Nursing?   3
What Are the Functions of Nurses?   8
A Conceptual Framework for Nursing   10

## 2. Personal Systems   19
Concept of Perception   20
Concept of Self   26
Concept of Growth and Development   29
Concept of Body Image   31
Concept of Space   34
Concept of Time   40

## 3. Interpersonal Systems   59
Concept of Human Interactions   59
Concept of Communication   62
Concept of Transactions   80
Concept of Role   89
Concept of Stress   95

## 4. Social Systems — 113

Concept of Organization   116
Concept of Authority   122
Concept of Power   126
Concept of Status   129
Concept of Decision Making   130

## 5. A Theory of Goal Attainment — 141

Philosophical Assumptions   143
Major Concepts in the Theory   144
Propositions   149
Boundaries of the Theory   149
Testing the Theory   150
Hypotheses   156
A Schematic Diagram of the Theory (Figure 5.3)   157

## 6. Application of a Theory of Goal Attainment in Nursing — 163

Goal-Oriented Nursing Record   164

## Index — 179

# A Theory for Nursing

# 1
# A Conceptual Framework for Nursing

Most individuals begin life as members of a group such as the family. Within the family, people learn ways of meeting their basic needs through interactions as members of a group. Through perceptions of the environment and through verbal and nonverbal communication, individuals engage in multiple interactions with family members and friends. Some of these interactions lead to transactions. Transactions are defined as purposeful interactions that lead to goal attainment. In nursing goals are achieved through nurse-client interactions when there is mutual goal setting by nurse and client, when both parties explore the means to achieve the goal and agree on the means, and when both exhibit behavior that moves toward goal attainment. The outcomes of transactions are satisfactions in performing activities of daily living, success in performing activities in one's usual roles, and achievement of immediate and long-range goals. Generally, human beings function in roles in a variety of groups such as the family and peer groups.

The artificial boundaries of nursing are individuals and groups interacting with the environment. Nurses function in their roles in a variety of health care environments. The domain of nursing is described by defining nursing, by outlining goals for nursing, by reviewing the functions of nurses, and by analyzing the values of the nursing profession.

## What Is Nursing?

Nursing is perceiving, thinking, relating, judging, and acting vis-à-vis the behavior of individuals who come to a nursing situation. A nursing situation is the immediate environment, spatial and temporal reality, in which nurse and client establish a relationship to cope with health states and adjust to changes in activities of daily living if the situation demands adjustment. Nursing is defined as a process of action, reaction, and interaction whereby nurse and client share information about their perceptions in the nursing situation. Through purposeful communication they identify specific goals, problems, or concerns. They explore means to achieve a goal and agree to means to the goal. When clients participate in goal setting with professionals, they interact with nurses to move toward goal attainment in most situations. Several characteristics of this concept of nursing as a process of human interactions leading to goal attainment have been identified (Peplau, 1952; Orlando, 1961; Nightingale, 1859; Rogers, 1970; King, 1971; Levine; 1975).

### CHARACTERISTICS OF NURSES

An understanding of the ways that human beings interact with their environment to maintain health is essential for nurses; this enables these professionals to promote health, to prevent disease, and to care for ill or disabled people. For example, a person admitted to a hospital is called a patient. This person can be observed in the role of mother when her children visit and in the role of wife when her husband visits. These interactions show the patient's role in her family. The patient may participate in the art guild in the community in the role of artist. The person functions in a variety of roles but in the hospital is perceived in the role of patient.

Here are several ways health can be promoted:

1. Nurses who function in well-baby clinics offer health guidance and information to mothers, and together they set goals for immunizations to prevent disease and promote growth and development
2. Nurses who function in ambulatory care settings observe and measure health states of people with chronic disease such as diabetes, and through mutual goal setting help individuals maintain a functional state of health and prevent complications.
3. Nurses who function in community agencies for health assessment of

the elderly engage in mutual goal setting to help older individuals function in their usual roles.
4. Nurses who teach parent classes offer information for expectant parents to prepare them for the birth of a child.

There is some kind of goal setting in each nursing situation. Goal setting depends upon the client population to be served and the specific events that bring individuals to health care systems in which nurses function. Nurses who provide care for individuals who are hospitalized because of illness, disease, or disability help them set goals and move toward achieving them. In the hospital, the nurse brings self to the role. The nurse also brings special knowledge, skills, and professional values to provide nursing care for patients.

Nurses help individuals and groups when they have some interference or disturbance in their health state, cannot help themselves, and may be hospitalized. Nurses interact with patients in hospitals to gather information systematically about past events and current signs and symptoms. Nurses listen to patients to gather information about their perceptions. Nurses and patients communicate information to each other so they can engage in mutual goal setting and can make decisions about the means to use to remove the disturbance or to solve the problem. This decision making requires collaboration with patients, other professionals, and family members.

Nurses use knowledge and skills to help individuals and groups cope with existential problems and learn ways of adjusting to changes in their daily activities. Many ambiguous cues, such as stressors, fears, anxieties, wants, and expectations, add to the complexity of nursing situations. The continuous discovery of knowledge in the natural and behavioral sciences and advancement in technologies have influenced changes in nursing. Continuous development of concepts and updating of psychomotor skills are essential for delivering quality nursing care to individuals and to groups. Nurses are concerned with human beings interacting with their environment in ways that lead to self-fulfillment and to maintenance of health.

## What Is the Goal of Nursing?

Since the turn of the century, nursing literature has described the goal of nursing. That goal is to help individuals maintain their health so they can function in their roles. The domain of nursing includes promotion of health, maintenance and restoration of health, care of the sick and injured, and care of the dying. A concept of health is essential for nurses if they are expected to help individuals achieve a goal of health.

## A CONCEPT OF HEALTH

Health has a high priority in the hierarchy of values in society. Health is a process of human growth and development that is not always smooth and without conflict. Illness may strike people at any age and in any socioeconomic group. Identity crises appear at different times in one's life: at puberty, marriage, vocational selection, pregnancy, and aging, to mention a few. Health relates to the way individuals deal with the stresses of growth and development while functioning within the cultural pattern in which they were born and to which they attempt to conform (King, 1971).

Illness and health have different meanings for individuals and groups in different cultures. It is known, however, that individuals have been endowed with particular genes that influence their life process. Although each human being is unique, facts are known about the ways in which most individuals grow, develop, cope with change, and solve some of life's problems (Gesell, 1952; Erikson, 1950; Kaluger and Kaluger, 1974). One of life's problems is the maintenance of a level of health that enables a person to perform activities of daily living in such a way that he leads a relatively useful, satisfying, productive, and happy life. This performance depends upon harmony and balance in each person's environment.

Some of the definitions of health proposed by individuals in and out of the health professions have alluded to attributes of health. Tempkin's (1953) historical survey of health as a concept indicated that, whether implicit or explicit, an ability to perform the functions of personal and social life has always been a part of this concept. Dubos (1961) noted that human life is a dynamic process and health is an adjustment of human beings to their total environment, which is always changing. He moved from a discussion of the abstract concept to the reality of life when he mentioned that freedom from disease and from life's struggles and problems is almost incompatible with the process of living. A review of some of the research conducted in the health field that might ultimately improve human existence leads one to appreciate that this abstract idea, health, is an aspiration and a goal that people continuously attempt to achieve (Koos, 1954; Duff and Hollingshead, 1968; Dubos, 1973).

The polarity between health and illness is almost a thing of the past. Individuals are viewing health as a functional state in the life cycle, and illness indicates some interference in the cycle. Health is important to individuals when factors arise that interfere with their performance of daily activities and maintenance of independence (Galdston, 1953; Seyle, 1956; Engel, 1960; Henderson, 1966; Dunn, 1961).

A person who is ill may be admitted to a hospital. Hospitalization increases a person's anxiety because of an actual or symbolic threat to one's self image (Schilder, 1951; Shontz, 1969; Smith, 1973; Grundemann, 1975). Patients fear mutilation and death. Patients cannot anticipate what will happen to them: clothes and personal belongings are removed, and the patient is placed in a passive role. These factors, and others, contribute to a loss of personal identity. There is a trend to change this hospital environment so that patients become actively involved in their care. The age of consumerism and the patient's bill of rights in hospitals have influenced some changes in hospital systems.

*Health is defined as dynamic life experiences of a human being, which implies continuous adjustment to stressors in the internal and external environment through optimum use of one's resources to achieve maximum potential for daily living.* Illness is defined as a deviation from normal, that is, an imbalance in a person's biological structure or in his psychological make-up, or a conflict in a person's social relationships. For example, disease is one kind of illness and for many years has been used as an indicator in reporting health statistics.

Human growth and development can be predicted for each age group in terms of characteristic patterns of behavior (Havighurst, 1953; Gentry and Paris, 1967; Mussen, Conger, and Kagan, 1974). The internal environment of human beings transforms energy to enable them to adjust to continuous external environmental changes. The developmental processes are manifested in verbal and nonverbal behaviors and can be observed, appraised, and in many instances measured to maintain health. Advances in nursing during the last 20 years have emphasized health teaching and health guidance as well as care of the ill (Sarosi, 1965; Vassalo, 1965; King, 1971).

**Health indicators.** Measurement of health continues to be a fundamental problem in the world. In 1957 a World Health Organization (WHO) expert committee recognized that there was no agreement on units of measurement of health (WHO, 1957).

Most measurements of health have been measurements of illness. One approach to measuring health has been to use health indicators such as vital statistics, morbidity and mortality figures, and nutrition data. Mortality rate is a crude indicator because it gives no data about social, economic, or emotional consequences of illness; it does not measure the effects of chronic diseases that are not primarily killers. Health services offered and accepted by individuals and environmental conditions within a community are a few of the factors associated with the health of a community.

Studies have supported the fact that standards of living are related to health. The fundamental problem of defining and measuring standards of living is that patterns of living throughout the world vary and that a single standard for all people does not seem feasible. However, there are some areas of living in which standards may be established, such as, what is the growth pattern in each cultural group around the world. Knowledge is available to measure growth in terms of nutrition, environmental factors such as clean air, accidents in the home, and social support systems related to health (Croog, Lipson, and Levine, 1972; Caplan, 1974; MacElveen, 1977).

The most recent work by the World Health Organization and the International Epidemiological Association has defined measurements of levels of health to include the incidence and prevalence of specific diseases and syndromes, measurements of physical and mental conditions, as well as social functions of individuals and population groups and their attitudes toward health and health-related activities. "Measurable variables are grouped under headings; measurements of ill health, measurements of need and demand for medical care, measurements of the use of health services and measurements of effectiveness and efficiency of health services and programs" (WHO, 1979, p. 9).

It is reasonable to assume that the events and situations that prevent illness are not necessarily identical with those factors that promote health. The factors responsible for health and illness must first be identified and measured. Since health and illness are interpreted as dimensions in the life events of a human being, the common factors that act in both should be isolated. Nurses are in a position to use epidemiological methods to identify factors in communities that relate to promotion of health and prevention of illness. They can use descriptive information to formulate hypotheses and test them in natural situations. If the attributes that are essential for human beings to function in their roles in social systems can be identified, then methods can be used to measure the health of individuals and communities.

A half century ago, most people recognized symptoms of illness because they were infectious and often debilitating. Today's longer life span has introduced concomitant proneness to chronic illness, which may be slow and insidious. In the United States, young people have been exposed to methods of health promotion (immunization, preschool physical and dental examinations, school hearing and sight programs, health teaching) as part of the total educational program in most school systems. One would expect that the young would have different perceptions of health than older persons in society, since their experiences have been different from those of their parents.

Popular magazines and newspapers impart information about health, illness, and new treatments. These sources of information, plus television and advertising, have contributed to changes in people's concept of health. Today people appear to want health information. If health information is to be effective, it must be communicated in such a way as to motivate each person to understand it and then to use it. Health education programs will increase their effectiveness if they are designed both to give the people what they want and to correlate this information with what epidemiological studies have shown are essential factors for health. Decisions must be based on a plan that combines the goals of the people with the facts that promote health. How can individuals be motivated to use information to promote health? The way people perceive health will depend on their past experiences, the environment in which they have lived, and their concept of health. Beliefs and rituals have a very important place in various societies, especially those that deal with crises of life, such as birth, death, marriage, and the ceremonial movement from one age group to another. Health professionals, overtly and covertly, exert some influence on a culture's notion of health, especially in teaching individuals ways to cope with change and to maintain and improve their health (Knutson, 1965; Leininger, 1978; White, 1977).

As methods of measurement continue to be designed, validated, and used, the current arbitrary distinction between health and illness will be more pronounced. The available measurements used in reported studies have indicated a relationship between standards of living and health in a community and society.

**Nursing and health.** Nurses are the largest group of health professionals in the United States. In recent years, nurses have begun to focus on health assessments and on planning for health promotion in communities. The educational programs preparing the future generation of nurses have placed emphasis on health maintenance and health promotion. Historically, health has been an integral part of the goal orientation of nurses, whether or not it has always been explicitly stated (Smith, 1933; Taylor, 1934; Sleeper, 1952; ANA, 1955; ANA, 1965; ANA, 1978; ANA, 1980).

The emphasis on primary nursing care in hospitals will give nurses the opportunities to provide health teaching, guidance, and continuity of care for individuals who have some temporary interference with their daily activities (NCNA, 1977). Nurses have become actively involved in the delivery of primary health care. One of their responsibilities is the objective assessment of functional abilities and disabilities of individuals and groups and the purposeful planning of goal-directed activities for them.

The emphasis in American society on positive health, on exercise and recreation programs, and on goal-oriented and achievement values delineates two major problems for the health professions: first, the discovery of methods of helping individuals cope with changes in their health; second, the discovery of new knowledge about human transactions with environment that are conducive to maintaining healthy individuals and communities.

Human beings have three fundamental health needs: (1) usable health information at a time when they require it and are able to use it, (2) preventive care, and (3) care when they cannot help themselves. The perception of one's health may be different from the signs and symptoms one's behavior manifests to others. Nurses are in a position to assess what people know about their health, what they think about their health, how they feel about it, and how they act to maintain it.

A concept of health is an essential dimension of nursing and health care. The dynamics of nursing involves accuracy of the nurses' perceptions and of the individuals' perceptions of their health status. The transactions that are made with recipients of care and families may provide a measure of effectiveness of nursing care.

## What Are the Functions of Nurses?

Nurses provide an essential service to meet a social need. Nurses teach, guide, and counsel individuals and groups to help them maintain health. Nurses give care to individuals and groups who, when acutely and moderately ill, are usually hospitalized. Nurses give care to individuals who have chronic diseases and to those who need rehabilitation to help them use their potential ability to function as human beings. Nurses are partners with physicians, with families, and with paramedical groups in the coordination of a plan of health care for individuals and groups.

Facets of the service require nurses to be skillful in a variety of techniques. Two such skills, observation and measurement, are essential for gathering relevant and accurate information in a systematic way. The information from measurements is important for making decisions about a course of action. Knowledge, understanding, and ability to evaluate observations of behavior and physiological measurements are basic to performing the functions of a professional nurse. Many individuals may learn how to gather information. The interpretation of specific information to plan, implement, and evaluate nursing care is the function of the professional nurse. Nurses work with individuals and with groups in a variety of environments. Nurses are expected to integrate knowledge from natural and behavioral sciences and the humanities and to apply knowledge in concrete situations. These situations arise in the home, in community health agencies, in local, state, and federal government agencies, in school systems, in occupational health settings, in hospitals, in ambulatory care and outreach clinics, and in crises centers. The method used by most nurses to assess, plan, implement, and evaluate care is called nursing process (Yura and Walsh, 1978).

Nursing process has been taught in many nursing education programs and has been presented in continuing education programs. Nursing process has become the standard method used in most nursing situations. This process has identified and explained some of the essential functions of nurses, which are assessment of the patients health, formulation of a plan on the basis of the information gathered, implementation of a plan of action and evaluation of its effectiveness. Using this nursing process requires prior knowledge about human behavior generally and behavior under stress specifically. Use of the process assumes nurses have assessment skills, interview skills, and communication skills as they interact with individuals to gather information and to identify goals and the means to achieve them. Paradigms, models, and theories organize related concepts and provide approaches for gathering information essential for decision making in nursing situations. Information overload, constant change, and a highly complex technological world have made it difficult for professionals to decide on what knowledge and skills are essential for educating the professional of the future. Moreover, the explosion of knowledge presents a problem for professionals to keep their knowledge and skills updated.

For the past 20 years or more there has been an emergence of a systems approach to deal with changes and complexity in health care organizations. Some scientists who have been studying systems have noted that the only way to study human beings interacting with the environment is to design a conceptual framework of interdependent variables and interrelated concepts (von Bertalanffy, 1968; Wiener, 1967; Churchman, 1968; Howland, 1976). The conceptual framework in this book presents one way to design interrelated systems for nursing.

## A Conceptual Framework for Nursing

A basic assumption is made that the focus of nursing is the care of human beings. If the goal of nursing is concern for the health of individuals and the health care of groups, and if one accepts the premise that human beings are open systems interacting with environment, then a conceptual framework for nursing must be organized to incorporate these ideas. The schematic diagram in Figure 1.1 provides for the organization of open systems in a dynamic interacting framework (King, 1971). Concepts are identified within each of these systems and are described and defined in subsequent chapters. A brief overview of these systems begins to demonstrate interactions within and between them through the concepts selected.

### PERSONAL SYSTEMS

Individuals are called personal systems. This means that the nurse as a person is a total system and the patient as a person is a total system. Selected concepts identified as relevant for understanding human beings as persons are: (1) perception, (2) self, (3) body image, (4) growth and development, (5) time, and (6) space. Individuals form groups, and formation of groups creates another kind of human experience within interpersonal systems.

**Interpersonal systems.** Several kinds of interpersonal systems exist. For example, two interacting individuals are called dyads; three interacting individuals are called triads. Selected concepts that help one understand interactions of human beings are: (1) role, such as self in role of professional health care provider called nurse, or self in role of health care consumer called client or patient, (2) interaction, (3) communication, (4) transaction, and (5) stress. Small and large groups are also called

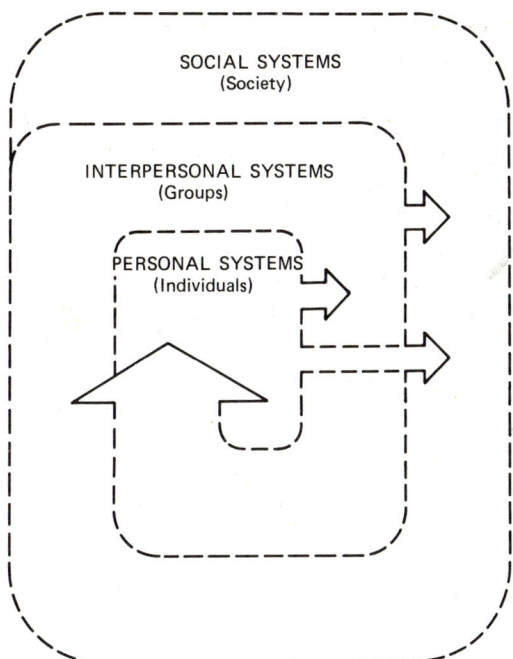

**Figure 1.1** A conceptual framework for nursing: dynamic interacting systems.

Reprinted with permission from I. M. King, *Toward a Theory for Nursing,* New York, John Wiley & Sons, 1971, p. 20.

interpersonal systems. Some of these groups with common interests and goals create another kind of human experience within a community or a society and are called social systems.

**Social systems.** The moving forces in nursing are imbedded in the dynamics of society in which the process of change alters the environment. Social forces are in constant motion within social systems, and the interplay of these forces influences social behavior, interaction, perception, and health. Fear, hope, anxiety, loneliness, and pain are a few of the behaviors confronted by nurses in their relationships with individuals in various nursing situations. Nurses are involved, too, on a day-to-day basis with change in degree of any one or more of the social forces.

A few examples of social systems in which nurses and consumers of health care interact are: (1) family systems, (2) religious or belief systems,

(3) educational systems, and (4) work systems. Health care systems are major social systems in the United States, such as hospitals, and public health agencies.

Several concepts provide knowledge to help nurses function in a variety of social systems. The few selected to help the beginning nurse function in health care systems are: (1) organization, (2) power, authority, status, (3) decision making, and (4) role.

One social system that influences nursing is the professional nursing organization, the American Nurses' Association (ANA). Within this organization, a code for nurses is promulgated and standards of nursing practice are disseminated for implementation by all nurses everywhere. Legal and ethical issues in nursing within health care systems are identified by the ANA, and positions are taken on critical issues affecting the profession. Within this structure, the values of the profession are identified. The conceptual framework presented here and the proposed theory in Chapter 5 incorporate some of the values and standards of organized nursing.

**What are the values of organized professional nursing?** The conceptual framework proposed for nursing offers one way to organize complexity and variety in the nursing profession. The preamble of the Code for Nurses is quoted because it is directly related to the conceptual framework and some of the philosophical assumptions about human beings in this book.

> The Code for Nurses is based on belief about the nature of individuals, nursing, health, and society. Recipients and providers of nursing services are viewed as individuals and groups who possess basic rights and responsibilities, and whose values and circumstances command respect at all times. Nursing encompasses the promotion and restoration of health, the prevention of illness, and the alleviation of suffering. (ANA, 1976; reprinted with the permission of ANA)

A code demonstrates a profession's commitment, accountability, and responsibility to clients for a service deemed essential by society. The Code for Nurses, adopted by the American Nurses' Association in 1950 and revised periodically, imparts to nurses and to society the profession's expectations in ethical decision making. "The requirements of the Code may exceed but are never less than those of the law" (ANA, 1976, p. 1).

Values of the profession are expressed in the published *Standards of*

*Nursing Practice* (ANA, 1973). Measures to judge the competence of its members are provided by professional organizations. By using standards, the quality of nursing's services can be evaluated.

## Summary

Nurses play strategic roles in the process of human growth and development and in helping individuals cope with disturbances in their health. They have an essential role in community planning for the delivery of health services to the public. As professionals, nurses deal with behavior of individuals and groups in potentially stressful situations, pertaining to health, illness, and crises, and help people cope with changes in daily activities.

The goal of nursing is to help individuals and groups attain, maintain, and restore health. If this is not possible, nurses help individuals die with dignity. The major functions of nurses have been identified in the nursing process, which has become a standard method in most situations.

An awareness of the complex dynamics of human behavior in nursing situations prompted the formulation of a conceptual framework that represents personal, interpersonal, and social systems as the domain of nursing. Selected concepts are identified within each of these three dynamic interacting open systems.

This framework indicates that human beings are the focus for nursing. Each of the dynamic interacting systems is artificially separated in the next three chapters for the purpose of presenting concepts basic to understanding each system and their relationships. The stage of development of each concept varies with different phases of knowledge.

Concepts are used to formulate conceptual frameworks and are also the building blocks for theory development. The major part of this book presents the development of concepts in a conceptual framework from which a theory for nursing was derived.

## Bibliography

Abramson, J. H., The Cornell Medical Index as an Epidemiological Tool, *Journal of American Public Health,* February 1966, 287–297.

American Nurses' Association, Professional Nursing Defined, *American Journal of Nursing,* 37(5), May 1937, 518.

American Nurses' Association, The Biennial, *American Journal of Nursing*, 46(11), November 1946, 728-746.

American Nurses' Association, ANA Board Approves a Definition of Nursing Practice, *American Journal of Nursing*, 55(12), December 1955, 1474.

American Nurses' Association, First Position Paper on Education for Nursing, *American Journal of Nursing*, 65(12), December 1965, 106-111.

American Nurses' Association, ANA Convention, '78, *American Journal of Nursing*, 78(7), July 1978, 1231-1246.

American Nurses' Association, ANA Convention—The 80's: Decade for Decision, *American Journal of Nursing*, 80(7), July 1980, 1317-1332.

American Nurses' Association, *Code for Nurses with Interpretative Statements*, American Nurses' Association, Kansas City, 1976.

American Nurses' Association, *Standards of Nursing Practice*, American Nurses' Association, Kansas City, 1973.

Batey, M. V., Conceptualization: Knowledge and Logic Guiding Empirical Research, *Nursing Research*, 26(5), September-October 1977, 324-329.

Beckstrand, J., The Notion of a Practice Theory and the Relationship of Scientific and Ethical Knowledge to Practice, *Research in Nursing and Health*, 1(3), October 1978, 1-36.

Beckstrand, J., The Need for a Practice Theory as Indicated by the Knowledge Used in the Conduct of Practice, *Research in Nursing and Health*, 1(4), December 1978, 75-79.

Benoliel, J. Q., The Interaction between Theory and Research, *Nursing Outlook*, 26(2), February 1977, 108-113.

Broderick, M. E., and Ammentorp, W., Information Structures: An Analysis of Nursing Performance, *Nursing Research*, 28(2), March-April 1979, 106-110.

Caplan, G., *Support Systems and Community Mental Health*, Behavioral Publications, New York, 1974.

Carper, B. A., Fundamental Patterns of Knowing in Nursing, *Advances in Nursing Science*, 1(1), October 1978, 13-23.

Carper, B. A., "The Ethics of Caring," *Advances in Nursing Science*, 1(3), April 1979, 11-19.

Chagnon, M., Audette, L. M., Lebrun, L., and Tilquin, C., A Patient Classification System by Level of Nursing Care Requirements, *Nursing Research*, 27(2), March-April 1978, 107-113.

Churchman, C. W., *The Systems Approach*, Dell, New York, 1968.

Croog, S., Lipson, A., and Levine, S., Help Patterns in Severe Illness: The Roles of Kin Network, Non-Family Resources and Institutions, *Journal of Marriage and the Family*, February 1972, p. 32.

Curtin, L. L., The Nurse as Advocate: A Philosophical Foundation for Nursing, *Advances in Nursing Science*, 1(3), April 1979, 1-10.

Dubos, R., *Mirage of Health*, Doubleday, Garden City, New York, 1961.

Dubos, R., *Man Adapting*, Yale University Press, New Haven, 1973.

Duff, R., and Hollingshead, A., *Sickness and Society*, Harper & Row, New York, 1968.

Dunn, H., *High Level Wellness,* R. J. Beatty, Arlington, Virginia, 1961.
Engel, F., A Unified Concept of Health and Disease, *Perspectives in Biology and Medicine,* Vol. III, Summer 1960, pp. 459-485.
Erikson, E., *Childhood and Society,* Norton, New York, 1950.
Fawcett, J., The What of Theory Development, in *Theory Development: What, Why, How,* National League for Nursing, New York, 1978, 17-33.
Fawcett, J., The Relationship between Theory and Research: A Double Helix, *Advances in Nursing Science,* 1(1), October 1978, 49-62.
Fromm, E., *The Art of Loving,* Bantam Books, New York, 1963.
Galdston, I., *The Epidemiology of Health,* Health Education Council, New York, 1953.
Gebbie, K. M., and Lavin, M. A., *Classification of Nursing Diagnosis,* Mosby, St. Louis, 1975.
Gentry, E., and Paris, L. M., Tools to Evaluate Child Development, *American Journal of Nursing,* 67(12), December 1967, 2544-2545.
Gesell, A., *Infant Development,* Harper & Row, New York, 1952.
Gordon, M., Nursing Diagnoses and the Diagnostic Process, *American Journal of Nursing,* 76(8), August 1976, 1298-1300.
Grundemann, B., The Impact of Surgery on Body Image, *The Nursing Clinics of North America,* 10(4), December 1975, 635-642.
Hardy, M. E., Theories: Components, Development, Evaluation, *Nursing Research,* 23(2), March-April 1974, 100-107.
Hardy, M. E., Evaluating Nursing Theory, in *Theory Development: What, Why, How,* National League for Nursing, New York, 1978, 75-86.
Hardy, M. E., Perspectives on Nursing Theory, *Advances in Nursing Science,* 1(1), October 1978, 37-48.
Havighurst, R., *Human Development and Education,* McKay, New York, 1953.
Henderson, V., *The Nature of Nursing,* Macmillan, New York, 1966.
Howland, D., An Adaptive Health System Model, in *Health Research: The Systems Approach,* edited by H. Werley, A. Zuzich, Zajkowski, M., and Zagornik, D., Springer, New York, 1976.
Jacobs, M. K., and Huether, S. E., Nursing Science: The Theory Practice Linkage, *Advances in Nursing Science,* 1(1), October 1978, 63-73.
Kaluger, G., and Kaluger, M., *Human Development: The Span of Life,* Mosby, St. Louis, 1974.
King, I. M., *Toward a Theory for Nursing,* John Wiley & Sons, New York, 1971.
Knutson, A., *The Individual, Society and Health Behavior,* Russell Sage Foundation, New York, 1965.
Koos, E., *The Health of Regionville,* Columbia University Press, New York, 1954.
Leininger, M., *Transcultural Nursing: Concepts, Theories and Practices,* John Wiley & Sons, New York, 1978.
Leininger, M. (ed), *Transcultural Health Care Issues and Conditions,* Davis, Philadelphia, 1976.
Levine, M., *Introduction to Clinical Nursing,* Davis, Philadelphia, 1975.

MacElveen, P. A., Social Networks, in Longo, D., Williams, R. (eds.), *Clinical Practice in Psychosocial Nursing,* Appleton-Century-Crofts, New York, 1977.

Mussen, P. H., Conger, J. J., and Kagan, J., *Child Development and Personality,* Harper & Row, New York, 1974.

Newman, M. A., Nursing's Theoretical Evolution, *Nursing Outlook,* 20(7), July 1972, 449–453.

Nightingale, F., *Notes on Nursing,* Dover, New York, 1969. From original American publication, 1860.

Nursing Clinics of North America, *Symposium on Primary Nursing,* 12(2), June 1977, 1–255.

Nursing Clinics of North America, *Symposium on Bioethical Issues in Nursing,* 14(1), March 1979, 1–91.

Nursing Clinics of North America, *Symposium on the Implementation of Nursing Diagnoses,* 14(3), September 1979, 483–569.

Nursing Theory—Conference Group, *Nursing Theories,* Prentice-Hall, Englewood Cliffs, New Jersey, 1979.

Orlando, I. J., *The Dynamic Nurse–Patient Relationships,* Putnam's, New York, 1961.

Peplau, H. E., *Interpersonal Relations in Nursing,* Putnam's, New York, 1952.

Rogers, M. E., *An Introduction to the Theoretical Basis for Nursing,* Davis, Philadelphia, 1970.

Sarosi, G., On the Nature of Nursing and the Phenomenon of Man's Health, *Nursing Science,* 3(4), August 1965, 306.

Schilder, P., *The Image and Appearance of the Human Body,* International Universities Press, New York, 1951.

Seyle, H., *The Stress of Life,* McGraw-Hill, New York, 1956.

Shontz, F., *Perceptual and Cognitive Aspects of Body Experience,* Academic Press, New York, 1969.

Sigman, P., Ethical Choice in Nursing, *Advances in Nursing Science,* 1(3), April 1979, 37–52.

Sleeper, R., What Kind of Nurse, *American Journal of Nursing,* 52(7), July 1952, 282.

Smith, C., Body Image Changes after Myocardial Infarction, *The Nursing Clinics of North America,* 8(4), December 1973, 663–668.

Smith, M., A Concept of Nursing, *American Journal of Nursing,* 33(6), June 1933, 565.

Stenberg, M. J., Ethics as a Component of Nursing Education, *Advances in Nursing Science,* 1(3), April 1979, 53–61.

Taylor, E., Of What Is the Nature of Nursing? *American Journal of Nursing,* 34(5), May 1934, 476.

Tempkin, O., What Is Health? Looking Backward and Ahead, in *Epidemiology of Health,* edited by Iago Galdston, Academy of Medicine, Health Education Council, New York, 1953, p. 21.

Vassalo, C., A Concept of Health, *Nursing Science,* 3(4), August 1965, 236–242.

von Bertalanffy, L., *General Systems Theory,* Braziller, New York, 1968.

White, E., Giving Health Care to Minority Patients, *Nursing Clinics of North America,* 12(1), March 1977, 27–39.

Wiener, N., *The Human Use of Human Beings,* Avon, New York, 1967.

World Health Organization, *Measurement of Levels of Health,* Technical Report Series No. 137, Geneva, Switzerland, 1957.

World Health Organization, *Measurement of Levels of Health,* WHO Regional Publications European Series No. 7, Copenhagen, Denmark, 1979.

Yura, H., and Walsh, M., *The Nursing Process,* Appleton-Century-Crofts, New York, 1978.

# 2
# Personal Systems

The world of experience is a personal world in which human beings actively process information from the environment. Individuals organize and categorize their human experiences by processing selective inputs through the senses. The categories (concepts) help persons relate past experiences to present events and give meaning and stability to their world. It is through perception that an individual comes to know self, to know other persons, and to know objects in the environment.

The focus of the conceptual framework is individuals interacting with other persons in a variety of social systems. However, in this chapter concepts have been developed with primary emphasis on knowledge that helps one understand individuals. The concepts of perception, self, growth and development, body image, time and space were selected as relevant knowledge for nurses to learn about human beings. For example, an individual's perceptions of self, of body image, of time and space influence the way he or she responds to persons, objects, and events in his or her life. As individuals grow and develop through the life span, experiences with changes in structure and function of their bodies over time influence their perceptions of self.

Individuals are characterized as social beings who are rational and sentient. Through language human beings have found a symbolic way of communicating thoughts, actions, customs, and beliefs. Persons exhibit some common characteristics, such as the ability to perceive, to think, to feel, to choose between alternative courses of action, to set goals, to select the means to achieve goals, and to make decisions. These characteristics indicate that human beings are reacting beings.

In the process of human interactions individuals react to persons, events, and objects in terms of their perceptions, expectations, and needs. Reactions occur in the perceptual milieu of the individuals who are interacting. In other words, persons react to each other's perceptions of the situation and to their own expectations of individuals and objects in the environment. Individuals react as total human beings to their experiences, which are viewed as a flow of events in time.

Individuals are time-oriented beings. Human beings have roots in past experiences, and their awareness of the present influences predictions of the future. Time is an irreversible process in life, yet the minds of individuals can recall past events, can make decisions in the present on the basis of past experiences, and can plan to achieve goals in the future on the basis of the past and present. Human acts, the behavior of individuals, are extensions in time and space, and depict various levels of complexity.

The perceptions, judgments, actions and reactions of human beings will determine the transactions they make in particular situations. If nurses are expected to have some understanding of human behavior in order to help people stay healthy and cope with interferences in their health, knowledge of perception is essential. Several concepts are described and defined that will help nurses understand persons as open systems: (1) perception, (2) self, (3) growth and development, (4) body image, (5) time, and (6) space.

## Concept of Perception

Images, percepts, sensory experiences, and concepts provide some basis for assuming that human beings have a higher mental process than other animals, and this belief is seen as a reflection of human ideas, memory, and cognition. Sensory experiences provide individuals with the raw data that helps them form particular and universal ideas as a way of knowing about their world.

Perception is each human being's representation of reality. It is an awareness of persons, objects, and events. Although one presupposes that human beings live in the same world and have some common experiences, individuals differ in what they select to enter their perceptual milieu. The perceptual tools, sensory (functioning sense organs) and intellectual (brain processes), vary from person to person. One's perception is related to past experiences, to concept of self, to biological inheritance, to educational background, and to socioeconomic groups.

Theoretical points of view in perception have influenced the research over the years (Weintraub and Walker, 1966). Several points of view support the idea that intact nervous systems and sensory systems are essential for persons to perceive the behavior of human beings and objects in the environment. For example, Gibson (1966) noted that perception depends on sensory experiences. He described perceptual systems as ways of gathering information from the environment.

The Gestaltists postulated that there is a relationship between the experience of an event, person, or object and the representation of it in the brain. This school of thought described wholeness as the configuration of a thing as it appears to a person. Lewin's theory supported these Gestalt ideas and noted that the perception of individuals organizes the field. His field theory indicated that persons described experiences as they appear to be, and the field included that which was directly experienced (Lewin, 1951).

Brunswick is known for his contribution to the theory of probabilistic functionalism. He indicated that people can seldom perceive all aspects of stimuli, and so they attend to cues and make judgments on the basis of incomplete information. He noted there was some uncertainty in predicting behavior from perceptual input (Brunswick, 1955).

More recent explorations in "person perception" view perception as an expression of the total human being with purpose, motives, and goals influencing what and how one perceives (Taguiri and Petrullo, 1958; Laing, Phillipson, and Lee, 1966).

Bruner's theory, for example, stated that a person categorizes input from sensory experiences and this categorization depends on the person's past experiences (Bruner & Krech, 1968). Klein notes two major approaches to the current movement in perception: (1) based on Gibson's work (1969), perception coordinates sensory input with environment, and (2) "person perception" deals with purpose, goals, and interests. Klein expressed concern for the limitation of information-processing models of perception reflected in input–output relationships. He believed that perception is part of a person's growth and development, which is influenced by and responsive to goals and needs. Perception, as an element in cognitive growth, should not be studied as an entity in itself (Klein, 1970, pp. 4–10).

Ittleson and Cantril characterized a transactional approach to perception in three ways: (1) the facts of perception always present themselves through concrete individuals dealing with concrete situations; (2) perceiving is done by a person from his own position in time and space and is based on past experience and present needs and values; (3) externalization is the term used to describe an individual who creates his own world by attributing certain parts of his experience to a world that he believes exists apart from that experience (Ittleson and Cantril, 1954,, p. 2). Some of the common characteristics of perception are suggested, which help one define the term.

## CHARACTERISTICS OF PERCEPTION

Prior to discussion of some of the characteristics of perception, a brief overview offers one approach for developing concepts. One of the methods used for conceptual analysis is an approach described in *Thinking with Concepts* (Wilson, 1963). Wilson suggests several techniques that will help one gain some precision in identifying defining characteristics of a concept. This approach is illustrated in nursing (Forsyth, 1980).

The major technique used in developing concepts in this book has been a review of the literature in nursing and related fields to identify characteristics of the concept. From this information, an operational definition of the concept is formulated and application to nursing situations is presented.

**Perception is universal.** All persons perceive other individuals and objects in the environment, and these experiences provide information about the world. Through these experiences, individuals form categories of the concrete world, and these abstractions are called concepts. For example, a person learns about a tree when he verifies his perceptions of the characteristics of a tree. The characteristics are leaves, branches, roots, trunk. The concrete elements form a concept called *tree*. This concept or category, which represents something in the environment, is stored in one's memory. Having formed a concept of tree, any future encounters with tree gives meaning to one's perceptions.

Although each human being is unique, individuals have similar equipment, such as the senses, with which to perceive the environment. A group of people may observe the same event but each person may perceive it differently. For example, a number of individuals may participate in the same group session and each leave with entirely different perceptions than other members of the group.

**Perception is subjective, personal, and selective for each person.** Perceptions are selective as each person permits some stimuli to enter from the environment. Experiences in each person vary in spatial-temporal relationships, in the integrity of the nervous system and/or disturbance in it, in the level of the person's development, and in the context or situation in which perceptions are experienced. Therefore, one cannot assume that each person in a situation perceives the events similarly. Perceptions are based on each person's background of experiences, which make them uniquely personal until communicated to others.

**Perception is action oriented in the present.** One views the world from information that is available. Perceptions are influenced by current interests, needs, and future goals. Human beings are in a continuous state of active participation in a perceptual milieu. Awareness of past events, values, and needs serve as organizing factors in one's perceptions. Role and status in the family, in the world of work, and in recreation influence perceptions of individuals. Perception and learning are interrelated concepts. What one knows influences perception and perception in turn enhances cognitive learning (Allport, 1955; Bruner, 1973).

**Perception is transactions.** Ittleson and Cantril indicate that all individuals enter a situation as active participants, and their existence in the interaction will affect their identity. Here is their description of the man-environment perspective:

> ... first, the facts of perception always present themselves through concrete situations. They can be studied only in terms of the transactions in which they can be observed. Second, within such transactions, perceiving is always done by a particular person from his own unique position in time and space and with his own combination of experience and needs. Perception always enters into the transactions from the unique personal behavioral center of the perceiving individual. Third, within the particular transaction and operating from his own personal behavioral center, each of us, through perceiving, creates for himself his own psychological environment by attributing certain aspects of his experience to an environment which he believes exists independent of the experience. (Ittleson and Cantril, 1954, p. 2)

Ittleson and Cantril named the above three features of perception externalization and viewed this label as a characteristic of perception. Furthermore, they identified two characteristics when they discussed perception as transaction, that is, taking place in a particular environment, and perception as unique to each person. From these characteristics and those identified in the literature, a definition of perception is derived.

## DEFINITION OF PERCEPTION

Perception is a process of organizing, interpreting, and transforming information from sense data and memory. It is a process of human transactions with environment. It gives meaning to one's experience, represents one's image of reality, and influences one's behavior.

It is essential for nurses to have a knowledge of perception if they are to assess, interpret, and plan for a client's identification and achievement of goals that maintain health. This concept is essential to an understanding of persons as systems and of the influence perceptions have on human interactions. It is a basic concept in the framework suggested for nursing and is a major concept in a theory of goal attainment presented in this book.

## APPLICATION OF PERCEPTION TO NURSING

Perception is a very important concept for nurses to develop as it is the basis for gathering and interpreting information. A subjective factor in perception, called *set*, was demonstrated in early studies of clinical inferences in nursing (Kelley and Hammond, 1964). For example, if one nurse hears another nurse report on the "uncooperative patient in the unit" and on another patient who is very "cooperative," a set may be established, and nurses may respond to those two patients in terms of the set rather than in terms of trying to assess the perceptions of both to determine any concerns or problems. *Stereotyping* is a facet of perception that needs exploration. If one has a *stereotyped* image of a supervisor as a person who is always looking over one's shoulder, then behavior toward that person will be affected. A *halo* effect is another facet of perception that influences behavior.

Perception may be distorted by high emotional states such as anger, fear, love. Emotions may partially close one's perceptual field and, thus, restrict the cues one allows to enter the perceptual field. An important element in nurse–patient interactions is accurate perception of each by the other. This accurate perception is a first step toward mutual goal setting and toward exploring means to move toward those goals.

Perceptual accuracy is important in nurse–client interactions. It begins with a nurse's initial assessment of a patient's intact sensory system, interference in any of the senses, the chronological age, the developmental level of patients, sex, and education. Drug and diet history gives information that may alert a nurse to elements that may influence a hospitalized patient's perceptions. Nurses ask patients to discuss their reasons for being in the hospital to get some idea of the patients' perceptions of what is happening to them.

Nurses need to be aware of the factors that influence their perceptions in patient care settings and of inferences that are made about patients on the basis of a few behavioral cues. One study showed that nurses' inferences of suffering differ according to their cultural and socioeconomic background, age, and diagnosis of patients (Davitz, 1969).

It is essential for nurses to assess the patients' stress, potential anxiety, needs, and readiness for learning about what is happening to them. Assessment of sensory and nervous systems will allow detection of any interference with a patient's perceptual system, and will allow the nurse to plan care according to the nurse's interpretations of the information gathered.

An overview of selected studies shows the relevance of this concept of perception to nursing. Many nursing functions involve human perceptions. Several studies in nursing have shown that patients' past experiences have influenced their perceptions in present situations (Bruegel, 1971; Joelson and Joelson, 1972; Johnson, 1972). For example, preoperative teaching of hospitalized adults provides information for patients and helps them understand why deep breathing, moving around, and coughing are beneficial in their postoperative recovery. One study found that children react more favorably to temperature taking when they had some "cognitive specific information" given to them by the nurse (McCaffery, 1971). Another study reported that increased body temperature changed people's perception of time (Alderson, 1974). Sensory deprivation and sensory overload have altered patients' perceptions, and some patients exhibit "deviant" behavior because of these sensory experiences.

Factors that may impair accuracy in perceptions are an internally altered nervous system, illness, drugs, alcohol, sensory stimulation, overload, or deprivation, use of defense mechanisms, and some personality factors. One of the early studies of nurse–patient interactions reported that the perceptions of nurses' needs and patients' needs were dichotomous (Whiting, 1959).

The environment in which nursing care is given may be perceived as sensory overload or sensory deprivation by patients. Either experience may cause perceptual distortion and less-than-normal expected behaviors in some environments. The temporal–spatial relationships in patient care environments may influence perceptions and, therefore, patients' behavior. If the illness for which the patient was hospitalized has caused disturbance in perception, the nurse must be alerted and plan care accordingly.

Perceptions may be altered in individuals when they experience a sensory loss, such as blindness or deafness. Another area of concern that may alter patients' perception is pain. These and other factors in the environment of health care systems may influence perceptions of the care giver and perceptions of the recipients of care. An important area of professional behavior is the need for nurses and patients to verify perceptions as they plan together to achieve their goals.

Perception is an essential concept in the framework and in the construction of a theory of goal attainment for nursing. It is also a basis for developing a concept of self.

## Concept of Self

Human beings can reflect on the past, speculate about the future, and express their ideas verbally and in writing. Customs and traditions have been preserved because they are passed from one generation to another through the written record. A cursory glance through history indicates that a search for the meaning of a concept of self has been going on for centuries. The saying "know thyself" is attributed to philosophers. Literature makes reference to self. For example, in Shakespeare's *Hamlet*, Polonius says: "to thine own self be true, and it follows as night the day, thou canst not then be false to any man."

Theologians, philosophers, and psychologists have asked the question: Who am I? Descartes answered: *Cogito, ergo sum* (I think, therefore I am). Knowledge of self is a key to understanding human behavior, because self is the way I define *me* to myself and to others. Self is all that I am. I am a whole person. Self is what I think of me and what I am capable of being and doing. Self is subjective in that it is what I think I should be or would like to be.

Self has been the subject of study in psychiatry, in counseling, in learning, in sociology, in medicine, and in nursing. Some characteristics have been identified that describe the nature of self.

### CHARACTERISTICS OF SELF

**Self is a dynamic individual.** The values and beliefs of individuals help them maintain some balance in their lives. When inconsistencies in beliefs tend to appear, the self tries to avoid them or clarify them. Each new experience tends to influence change in self.

**Self is an open system.** Self-preservation is innate in each person. However, the self is protected with artificial boundaries. The physical body, for example, is covered with skin for protection. Self is perceived in relation to another person and to objects in the environment. Interactions with relevant others give one a sense of self. Attitudes toward self are often reflected in attitudes toward others. Self is an integral part of a person's human experiences. If these experiences are positive, the self is enhanced; if negative, the self may need assistance.

**Self is goal-oriented.** The self is a complex and highly organized system that differentiates self from every other person. The self is the I that makes me what I am and what I appear to be. Each person is unique in genetic inheritance, in experiences, and in perceptions of the external world. In the process of growth and development, each person has acquired a system of values, needs, and goals that gives him or her an awareness of personal separateness; yet each person's value system recognizes the influence of significant others and their reactions to the self. Goal orientation directs activities toward fulfillment of self. Several writers have defined the concept of self.

## DEFINITION OF SELF

Rogers defines self as a person's interaction with the environment, which is influenced by feedback from interactions with others and which gives some consistent patterns of relationships of the *I* or the *me* (Rogers, 1961).

The *I*, the *me*, the *self*, the *person* are synonyms used in the search for some unity in experience. A personal system is a unified, complex whole, self who perceives, thinks, desires, imagines, decides, identifies goals and selects means to achieve them.

Jersild's definition of self includes many of the characteristics of self.

> The self is a composite of thoughts and feelings which constitute a person's awareness of his individual existence, his conception of who and what he is. A person's self is the sum total of all he can call his. The self includes, among other things, a system of ideas, attitudes, values and commitments. The self is a person's total subjective environment. It is a distinctive center of experience and significance. The self constitutes a person's inner world

as distinguished from the outer world consisting of all other people and things. The self is the individual as known to the individual. It is that to which we refer when we say "I." (Jersild, 1952, pp. 9–10)

This definition is accepted as a definition of self for the concept presented here.

## IMPLICATIONS FOR NURSING

Every nurse and client has a concept of self. Awareness of self helps one to become a sensitive human being who is comfortable with self and with relationships with others.

Consumers of health care are concerned about the dehumanization and depersonalization of individuals as they enter the health care systems. The environment of some hospitals may threaten the patient's selfhood. Some professionals remove all control and power for decision making about self and events from clients. Some policies in health care systems imply that the patient is not a rational human being during these experiences in life. For example, a patient may have been taking physician-prescribed medication at home for a year. Upon admission to a hospital, the same person is not allowed to have medicines in the room, and someone in the system administers the medicines to the patient.

When interference in self occurs, such as an identity crisis, a disturbance in physiology, or a rapid change in boundaries, a person may seek help from professionals. If the interference relates to health and an ability to function in social roles, the person may enter the health care system. Some individuals enter the system to have routine checks on their health status. Knowledge of self is evident in every nurse–client interaction. The clients' and the nurses' perceptions influence nursing care. If nurses are to help individuals they must have some understanding of how clients perceive self and current health status.

If nurses and other professionals interact with patients or clients as human beings, and let the individuals be themselves, even if they do not match the stereotype of the "good patient," nurses and patients would help each other grow in self-awareness and in understanding of human behavior, especially in stressful life experiences.

Each self is a whole person who grows and develops in a specific society. A concept of self is reflected in patterns of growth and development and in the structure and function of human beings.

# Concept of Growth and Development

Individuals and groups have been subjects of studies, and findings have been reported about the way human beings are born, grow, develop, age, and die. There have been a number of studies in the way individuals grow and develop through childhood, adolescence, and adulthood, and these have provided knowledge that enables health professionals to assess what is predicted as normal growth and development for all relatively normal newborns. These concepts are mentioned to show their relevance to a concept of self. Only highlights and summary statements are discussed, with references for further reading.

If one looks at old family picture albums, a concept of growth is readily apparent. One can see family resemblances from one generation to another. An observation can be made that people grow in height and in weight but the dynamics of development are not so easily detected in pictures. One can observe space and time transformations in photographs.

Several writers and professionals have influenced the discovery of knowledge about human growth and development. In the first few decades of the twentieth century, studies concentrated on the description of trends in cognitive and physical characteristics of children. Differentiation and alteration in physiological growth influence cognitive and behavioral development of human beings. The physical and chemical changes occurring in people determine the quantitative and qualitative phases of growth and development. Although individuals pass through specific experiences, there is a variation in the timetable for each individual. For example, a mother may say that Joan's first tooth erupted at 6 months but Betty's did not come until 8 or 9 months. John walked in less than 1 year, but Joe did not walk for 18 months. There are some normal values that predict growth, such as speech and walking. However, studies of adults and of those who are growing old have less predictive information. For example, menopause in women varies greatly. The mental capacity in some people at age 70 is as good as that in others at age 50.

Freud's psychoanalytic theory (1966) proposed four stages of development: (1) oral stage in infancy; (2) anal stage from 2–3 years; (3) phallic stage in preschool years; and (4) genital stage in adolescent. He noted that the source of behavior came from biological energy that can be directed in different ways.

Eight stages of growth and development were defined by Erikson

(1950). He noted that these stages proceeded in a more or less orderly sequence: (1) basic trust vs. mistrust; (2) autonomy vs. shame and doubt; (3) initiative vs. guilt; (4) industry vs. inferiority; (5) identity vs. identity diffusion; (6) intimacy vs. isolation; (7) generativity vs. self-absorption; and (8) integrity vs. disgust, despair. He believed that the family and the environment influenced the psychosocial development of individuals.

Piaget's theory (1964) identified cognition as an ability to reason, to think in a logical manner, and to conceptualize events in the environment. An individual is actively involved in exploring the environment. Piaget described four stages of development. From birth to 18 months, a child moves from uncoordinated motor activities to coordinated functions. After some weeks of hitting at toys, a child begins to move toys in different places in the space surrounding him. From 18 months to 7 years a child uses language and meanings of events to manipulate the environment, and some symbols have been developed. From 7–12 years, a child develops concepts and relations between words, such as John is taller than Joe. From 12 years on, formal operations begin, and a child employs deductive reasoning about events. The child can conceptualize things in the environment and can use abstract ideas and rules in problem solving.

Gesell (1952) believed that a child matured because of the development of the central nervous system. His charts for measuring growth and development have been widely used.

Developmental tasks in adulthood were described by Havighurst (1953). He believed that some tasks are mastered with physical growth; some tasks are achieved from society's expectations; some tasks are completed because of personal goals and values. These events are part of developing character and personality of self.

Several characteristics of growth and development have been identified.

## CHARACTERISTICS OF GROWTH AND DEVELOPMENT

**Growth and development include cellular, molecular, and behavioral changes in human beings.** Although these changes are continuously taking place, there is continuity and regularity due to anabolism and catabolism. Under normal circumstances there is order in growth and development, that is, patterns develop in people that are predictable but vary because of individual differences. The manner in which a person grows and develops is influenced positively and negatively by other people and objects in the environment.

**Growth and development are a function of genetic endowment, meaningful and satisfying experiences, and an environment conducive to helping individuals move toward maturity.** These factors influence a concept of self. Growth and development describe the processes that take place in people's lives that help them move from potential capacity for achievement to self-actualization.

This information is important for nurses to assess a patient's ability to perform functions associated with activities of daily living. The behavior exhibited by adults can sometimes be understood if the nurse has some knowledge of a client's background of growth and development. This knowledge is necessary to plan for health teaching, for care in the hospital, in the home, and in the community.

Age is the time measure of various stages of growth and development. It is a critical variable in any nursing situation because it defines for nurses and for patients the stage of their developmental tasks, and their responses to each other may be influenced by stages they have successfully achieved. Nurses who work with children and parents must have knowledge of growth and development to help parents and their children understand what is happening to them at various stages and especially when there is some disturbance in the normal process of living. The nurse may be the first professional to detect some interference in the growth and development pattern. When nurses know the patterns of growth and development they may use this knowledge to help adults through stressful periods in their lives. Nurses can understand the why of patients' behavior. This knowledge can help nurses predict situations and times of high risk for children and adults prone to accidents or disease. Knowledge of self and of the way people grow and develop helps nurses understand people who have a problem with body image, which is related to a concept of self.

# Concept of Body Image

Body image may be viewed as an integral component of growth and development, which in turn influences a concept of self. Body image is the picture one has of one's own body bound in space, which constitutes one aspect of the idea of *I*.

## CHARACTERISTICS OF BODY IMAGE

Body image is a very personal and subjective concept. It is acquired or learned in the process of growth and development. This is demonstrated in observations of the newborn who, through visual, auditory, tactile, and other sensory experiences, perceive toes and fingers and begin to sense the body boundary as separate from others. Each person's body is unique because each person has a unique genetic inheritance, differing experiences, and variety in environmental forces.

The dynamic characteristic can be seen in the development of body image through a lifetime. As experiences and perceptions change, body image changes. As a person redefines self, passing from one age group to another, identity is assessed, and body image may change. Individuals behave in terms of their perceptions of self, others, and situations; thus, persons have a concept of body image whether conscious or unconscious. It is a universal principle that individuals identify self in relation to their body appearance and others' reactions to them. This identification occurs in all cultures, age groups, both sexes, and all socioeconomic groups.

Because body image is a part of each stage of growth and development, sociocultural factors influence the standards against which body image is perceived. For example, emphasis on beauty products, on beauty pageants, on body beautiful, exerts some pressure or tension on a person's concept of his or her body.

For centuries great artists have depicted the human body and their personal image of it. Changes in body structure can be observed in these masterpieces. Body structure and functions are an integral part of understanding growth, development, self, and body image. Structure and functions of human beings studied in courses in anatomy and physiology give nurses knowledge that is essential for understanding patients.

## DEFINITION OF BODY IMAGE

Schilder defined body image as that idea a person forms in his mind about his own body; that is, the way in which one's body appears to self (Schilder, 1951). He described body image as tridimensional, physiological, psychological, and sociological. Several definitions agree with Schilder's and add that body image is both conscious and unconscious (Wapner and Werner, 1965; Fisher and Cleveland, 1968). Shontz added that body image is an integral part of a person's ego (Shontz, 1969).

Nurses have been writing about body image. Norris discussed body image as the constantly changing feelings and perceptions of one's body in space as different from others (Norris, 1970, p. 42). McCloskey noted that the concept included one's perceptions of body sensation, body functions, and mobility (McCloskey, 1976, p. 69). Gruendemann emphasized that body image is dynamic and changes with experiences. It is based on appearance, sensations, and the reactions of people to him. Gruendemenn, 1975, p. 636).

Body image is defined as a person's perceptions of his own body, others' reactions to his appearance, and is a result of others' reactions to self.

## IMPLICATIONS FOR NURSING

Throughout a person's life span, there are disturbances in his perception of self and his body image from threat, real or imagined, from trauma, and from loss of body parts. When these events occur, a person may be unable to cope with them and seek help from a professional in the health field. These disturbances are usually associated with crises in a person's life.

Some of the events relate to a diagnosis of a chronic disease, such as diabetes, paralysis, amputation of a leg, removal of a breast. It is the responsibility of the nurse to be aware of perceived threats to body image, to develop goals with the patient, and to plan for active participation in implementing the means to achieve goals.

Individuals with progressive neurologic and arthritic changes experience loss of function, which means loss of control and change in body structure and function. Nurses play an important role in assisting patients with body image distortions due to such things as mental disturbances or drug-related changes in body image and disfigurement from accidents, burns, or surgery. Nurses must examine their own feelings and attitudes toward individuals whose body image may become distorted. Nurses must be aware of the patient's perceptions of body changes and the influence on one's life style. Family members may need help from nurses to cope with changes in body image of a loved one because the person may be watching responses from family members to detect acceptance, rejection, pity, and anger. It is important to help patients maintain self-esteem and interact in ways that give them opportunities to make choices and exert some control over what is happening to them. Nurses must be aware that other concepts come into being in disturbances in body image, such as loss, separation, grief, and anger.

Several assessment tools have been published that assess changes in behavior in crisis situations. Roberts identified several phases the patient will pass through when body image disturbance is perceived as a crisis. The shock that accompanies the event is called the *impact phase*. Patients may exhibit anger, guilt, or despair, or they may use defense mechanisms such as denial or withdrawal to protect self. *Retreat phase* begins when the patient realizes what has happened. Whether or not patient perceptions of what is happening are accurate or distorted, the nurse must help the patient gather adequate information and seek participation in planning care (Roberts, 1976, p. 77).

In the third phase, which is *acknowledgment,* the patient may begin to discuss the situation, ask questions about what can be done and about when and how he can cope after leaving the hospital. For example, a patient with a colostomy may begin to look at the stoma and gradually be able to irrigate the colostomy. A woman may be able to glance at the incision resulting from a mastectomy. The nurse can help patients begin to look, to talk, to touch, and eventually to cry about what has happened. Through multiple interactions, nurses can plan with patients in setting goals that seem reasonable and are feasible. They may try several means to achieve goals, and this leads to a fourth phase, *reconstruction*. At this time, plans for discharge from the hospital are made and, if necessary, plans for continued patient teaching. Community resources are identified and their uses suggested to patient and family.

It is important for nurses to understand a concept of body image and alterations in that image. Nurses are the most constant individuals in the patient's environment and play a vital role in helping the patient when disturbances of body image have occurred.

## Concept of Space

Space is an essential component in an open systems framework. The concept was selected for inclusion within a personal systems framework because of its relationship to perception, body image, and the way individuals use space.

Philosophers, mathematicians, psychologists, and ethnologists have studied space. *Territoriality, proxemics,* and *personal space* are terms that have been used to describe space. Territoriality is the physical area that animals claim as their own and defend from predators. Ardrey (1966) discussed animal studies and territory, and noted that human beings have a need to acquire and defend their territory.

Hall (1959) agrees that, initially, territoriality described animal behavior, but the term has been extended to describe human behavior. War among nations is but one example of marking off physical space and defending it. A second term, *proxemics,* was coined by Hall (1963) to describe the use of space as an "elaboration of a culture." He noted that individuals have four ways of handling distance. Intimate distance is 6 to 18 inches; personal distance is $1\frac{1}{2}$ to 4 feet; social distance is 4 feet to 12 feet or more; public distance is 12 to 25 feet and over, but 30 feet around public figures. These distances change, depending upon persons' interactions, purposes, goals, knowledge, and situation. The use of space explains communication in various cultures (Hall, 1966).

Four types of territories in human societies were proposed by Lyman and Scott (1967). Space around the body is called *body territories. Interactional territories* are observed when people gather together to interact for a purpose. *Home territories* represent areas where those who frequently come to the place have control over the space. *Public territories* are areas where people have use of space, such as schools, but this space may be restricted to specific persons at designated times.

Watson's cross-cultural study of proxemic behavior (1970) examined the way in which people structure space in interactions. Thermal factors, touch, tone of voice, and sense of smell determined spacing.

A third term, *personal space,* is described as that invisible territory in which individuals place themselves. Sommer (1969) indicated that space described the way a person marked out an area to inhabit. He believed that personal space and interpersonal distance interact to influence the way persons distribute themselves. He noted a connection between space and status. For example, a person who is in a high position in the organization usually is allocated the larger and better space. Spatial norms exist in rules, spoken or unspoken, in organizations, such as the faculty dining room in a university, the board room in a corporation, the classroom with designated space for teacher and for learner.

Nurses have reported studies of space in relation to hospitalized patients. Allekian asked whether intrusion of territory and personal space was anxiety-provoking for hospitalized patients. She noted that anxiety was increased in patients who have their chair moved or removed from a certain space or their personal items moved around from drawer to drawer without permission. The most anxiety-producing event related to intrusion of personal space occurred when patients could feel the nurses' breath when nurses leaned over patients. Intrusion of patients' territory was seen as a decrease in patient control and identity (Allekian, 1973).

When individuals enter the hospital they are placed in the role of patient as defined by that institution. Their cues come from the building, the defined space for patients, and the behavior of nurses and physicians.

Stillman (1978) indicated that nurses can decrease the patient's anxiety by permitting the patient to make some decisions so that he has some control over his environment. For example, nurses should ask patients if they prefer the door to the room open or closed. When procedures are done for a patient that involve body contact, the nurse should explain the procedure to the patient. The patient's privacy should be protected, and discomfort should be minimized by performing procedures with skill and economy of time and energy. Possession of territory and protection of personal space give hospitalized patients a sense of security and identity.

Barnett (1972) discovered that touch, which can be perceived as an invasion of one's personal space, was misinterpreted 50 percent of the time by patients. Touch increases patients' anxiety. She suggested that when patients need to protect their personal space or territory, they had a lesser need for touch.

Trierweiler (1978) examined personal space and its meaning for the elderly. Aged individuals are spending more time in institutional settings rather than in their own homes. Sometimes there is overcrowding, and they have reduced personal space. Personal space in the elderly is related to one's identity as an individual, to one's control of environment, and to one's feeling of independence. Alterations in personal space lead to the older person's withdrawal and to antisocial behavior.

Personal space differs from territory in that boundaries in the former are not visible, whereas boundaries in the latter are fixed areas; personal space moves with the person. Hall (1963) defined proxemics related to spatial zones as intimate, social, personal, and public. Pluckhan (1968) believed that space influenced one's intrapersonal and interpersonal communication. Individuals communicate through the use of space and therefore personal space is individual and subjective.

## CHARACTERISTICS OF SPACE

**Space is universal.** All people have some concept of space. It exists everywhere and has no boundaries. Hall (1966) refers to space as an invisible and intangible bubble that extends self in space.

**Space is personal.** Space exists to the extent that it is perceived by each person and is, therefore, unique. The use of perception of space is rooted in cultures and communicated in behaviors learned through the culture. Spatial arrangements communicate role, position, and interactions with others. Marking off an area for self gives individuals a sense of security and identity. Space orients a person to his or her environment. The need for space varies with each person's needs. A person's arrangement of objects, such as furniture in an office, gives clues to that person's need for and use of space. Space is subjective and identifies what is *mine*. Spatial differences are individual, due to each person's perceptions. Space is unique to an individual and influenced by needs, past experiences, and culture.

**Space is situational.** Less space is provided for people in a crowded elevator than for those walking in a hallway. Crowding is tolerated more in cold weather than in hot. A person's space at work is usually less than his space at home. Each situation changes the need for and the way one uses space. A person's fears, anxieties, joys, and pleasures influence the need for space in situations. Spatial distance can be expanded or contracted depending on the nature of the relationship in each situation. In some settings, such as a hospital, a person's spatial needs are altered; the space is limited, the individual experiences are lessened. Some situations tend to bring people together and some tend to keep them apart. An individual's personal space is altered from one situation to another.

**Space is dimensional.** Space is a function of area (length times width), of volume, of distance, and of time. People with status in an organization are usually given large areas of space. Webster's defines space "as a system of one temporal and three spatial coordinates by which any physical object or event can be located."

**Space is transactional.** A person's use of space is based on his perception in a situation. The manner in which space is used communicates messages with different meanings in different cultures. Space determines the transactions between human beings and environment. The way in which people perceive space influences the way they will behave in certain spatial situations. Spatial distance increases with differences in status and decreases with increased interpersonal liking.

## DEFINITION OF SPACE

Space is defined as existing in all directions and is the same everywhere. In geometry, space is defined as an area made up of length times width.

Space is defined as the physical area called territory and by the behavior of individuals occupying space.

Defense of personal space can be observed by people's gestures, postures, and the visible boundaries they erect to protect their space from trespassers. Use of space and defense of space is nonverbal communication. The change in distance between people as they interact tends to communicate different messages to different people. Personal space is related to time, distance, area, volume, perception, and communication.

## APPLICATION TO NURSING

Knowledge of a concept of space is relevant for nurses to understand self in relation to personal space and then to assess the patient's perception of personal space. For example, when a person is admitted to a hospital, and placed in restricted space called patient's room and bed number, the person exhibits a need to mark off personal territory. However, personal space is often violated by all the hospital personnel who enter and leave that space, some who enter without asking permission and some who perform procedures without communicating the purpose for the invasion. Allekian's study (1973) showed that patients were annoyed when their territory was disturbed, such as when their beds were bumped and moved slightly or when the tables at their bedsides were rearranged or disturbed or when personal things were pushed out of the patients' reach and replaced with hospital equipment.

Nurses must be aware of the close distance that is involved when giving personal care to patients. Many procedures are performed in the intimate zone described by Hall (1963). Some patients may view touching as a comfort and a sign of caring while others may view it as a discomfort and a frightening sign. Patients are often transferred from one room to another and from one unit to another without an explanation and, thus, patients' space alterations may influence their sense of loss of identity and of security.

Intensive care units provide limited space for patients and restricted space within which the nurse must perform lifesaving functions. The lack of personal private space in such situations may influence patients' behavior.

Nurses should assess elements of patients' perception of personal space on admission to the hospital. An attempt to help patients organize their space may prevent undue anxiety and stress during hospitalization. Use of space communicates needs of patients and communicates caring by nurses. Observations of hundreds of patients in the recovery room demonstrated that patients tended to touch siderails upon regaining consciousness as though to establish contact with their spatial environment (Minckley, 1968). Where patients were close to each other, some would cover their faces with a sheet to provide less intrusion in their space. Patients wanted to know when they could return to "their" room.

Some behaviors that show negative reactions to an invasion of space are lowered eyes, rigidity, turning away from a person, and leaving the situation. Individuals need to arrange space to meet their needs. Alterations in patients' perceptions may alter their ideas of spatial needs. Placement of furniture in the patients' space, position of telephone, bedside stand, position of window curtains and personal belongings may influence patients' perceptions. When nurses take the time to ask questions to determine a patient's perception of personal space, the patient may feel a sense of identity.

Hospital space is regulated by laws, accrediting bodies, and policies. Many spaces are specialized, such as critical care, medical intensive care, emergency care. These environments are arranged to meet the physical needs of patients, and in their design, the personal space needs of patients and of nurses have been overlooked. Nurses seldom are members of hospital committees that design the space and its use.

Knowledge of personal space has not been applied to any great degree by nurses with patients, although observations indicate that the personal space of patients is being invaded. Nurses with knowledge of space can prevent some of the intrusions by exerting a greater control over the patient care environment. Nurses can facilitate appropriate draping of patients to prevent undue exposure of the body. In some instances, visitors may be restricted. Nurses can include in their assessment questions that will gather information about the patients' perception of personal space. Nurses can instruct other personnel to respect personal space of patients.

Nurses who understand cultural differences in patients will be aware of differences in their personal space. Nurses should also be aware of space distance as they interact with patients. Nurses should occupy space in patients' environment that communicates "I care," "I want you to participate in decisions." When entering the space of patients, nurses should explain their purpose for doing so. Nurses who are aware of their own perceptions of personal space and distance will be more conscious of these factors in patients.

The spatial–temporal dimensions in the life space of human beings must be given more recognition and emphasis in planning health care facilities and in the delivery of health care services. Although personal space is taken for granted in wellness and in performing activities of daily living, professionals must be aware of intrusions of personal space in times of illness.

Admission to a hospital may be perceived by patients as a territorial crisis. Patients attempt to defend their individuality, to control their environment, yet they feel their personal space is being invaded. Patients feel assignment to a room and a bed gives them some defined personal space in the system. Observations indicate that many patients begin to mark off their space and guard it.

Nurses are required to enter patients' personal space when giving direct nursing care. They can explain to the patient everything that will be done and how it will be done. Patients must be oriented to the space in the hospital so they have some idea of their total environment. Then they must have some orientation to the larger space surrounding their room. This orientation provides some sense of security about space for the patient.

Identity of self is related to personal space. The behaviors people exhibit when defending personal space indicate one way they try to maintain integrity. When individuals enter the health care system, they leave their own space and enter territory perceived as someone else's space. They are given restricted personal space within the system and have little control over it because professionals in caring for patients tend to invade their space, which may be for their benefit. The many diagnostic tests and procedures, the medications and treatments may be perceived by patients as invasion of their personal space and may add to their stress. Hospital policies are changing but not because planners have knowledge of space but because consumers are demanding changes. A concept of space is related to temporal dimensions in the world of reality.

## Concept of Time

Historically time was recognized as movement of the sun. Aristotle tried to define time within Greek philosophy as the before-and-after of events. Christians viewed time as linear, with events moving forward and not to be repeated. In the twentieth century, time and space are viewed as interrelated abstractions. Priestley (1964) noted that objects occupy space and that there would be no space if objects were nonexistent; if there were no changes in objects there would be no time. Orme noted that there is only one world of time "changing within itself only with space" (Orme, 1969, p. 147). Fraser (1972) believed time gave order and duration to events in the world.

Copernicus, an astronomer, proposed a concept of motion and its relation to time. Galileo, a physicist and astronomer, added acceleration to the idea of time. He was followed by Newton, who introduced the idea of absolute time that is continuous and sequential like a geometric straight line and independent of motion. Einstein's theory of relativity indicated that time is relative rather than absolute, that the rate of time is influenced by mass.

## TIME PERSPECTIVES

Studies have been conducted to explain biological time, which regulates the internal rhythm of human beings and which is called circadian rhythms, periodicity, and rhythmicity (Edelstein, 1972; Tom and Lanuza, 1976). These studies indicate that time is an important concept in nursing.

Some studies of psychological time, which is subjective or experiential, have shown that one person may perceive the same period of time as longer in duration than another person due to various kinds of events in which the person is involved (Ornstein, 1969). Time is not only the order of events, but the duration experienced by each person. Physical time tends to speed up with age.

For centuries time has been described by one school of thought as a cyclic concept and by another as a linear and irreversible concept measured by clocks and calendars. Another concept of time presented over the years has been a relational one, in that it connects past with present and future; it is sequential order or the organization of successive events.

Comments that occur everyday indicate that time is a part of everyone's daily living. What time is it? Can you wait one more minute? I'll be there in a second. How long will the class be in session? Do you have the time? Do we have time to spare before the meeting begins? These types of questions are asked everyday by someone in some place. The nature of time is complex and abstract. We can't touch it, see it, smell it, but we consistently and continuously talk about it and try to measure it with modern clocks and calendars.

As technology improves, so does the development of instruments to measure time. Time rules people's lives in a technological society. Time controls the workday of many individuals. For example, in a hospital, nurses have specific times to administer different kinds of medication to the patients, specific times to see to the patients' diagnostic tests, specific times for the performance of selected procedures, specific times to work and to stop work. Modern life in advanced societies is ruled by the clock.

Time is now, but the past is recognized by special days given to anniversaries such as birthdays, wedding dates, memorial days. In the United States great celebrations take place to mark the end of one year and the beginning of a "new" year on New Year's Eve.

## TIME AND COMMUNICATION

The way in which one values time will influence relationships with other people. In some cultures, waiting over an hour for a meeting is usual practice, whereas in other cultures waiting is a form of control or of status, such as waiting for an appointment with an employer, or waiting in a clinic to be seen by a physician.

Formal organizations such as industry, business, factories, and hospitals have organized the achievement of goals around a rigid time schedule. Some flexibility in scheduling in hospitals has been initiated within the past few years, but little or no importance has been given to the correlation between patients' biological rhythms and scheduling for tests, treatment, and surgery. Information about the way individuals perceive time may enhance communication in most situations.

Time is change. Nothing stands still; everything is in motion. When reflecting on living in the world one can never cease to wonder at the magnificence, the order of the universe, the flow of time. Time moves forward to infinity.

## CHARACTERISTICS OF TIME

All that has been written about time indicates that this concept is complex and abstract. Time is said to be relational, durational, and measurable. Time is ubiquitous and so it is universal. Time is the subjective perception of a succession of events from past to present to future. *Time is irreversible.*

**Time is universal.**  Inherent in the life processes is the rhythmic flow of events As the earth turns on its axis, day changes to night. As the earth moves around the sun, seasonal changes are noted. Plants, animals, and humans are known to have internal clocks that are influenced by patterns of things in the environment (Luce, 1971).

**Time is relational.** In this sense, time is individual and based on each person's uniqueness and perceptual milieu. Studies of time estimation demonstrated relativity in that time interval seemed longer when space was greater. Two observers at different distances from an event will see it at different times (Newman, 1976). Movement of time and the experience of time are related in that an interval of time that is filled with information seems short in duration. When intervals are unfulfilled, time seems longer. People's immediate experience with time is related to the sequence of events. People perceive time as one event following another, which makes time continuous. If life consisted of only instants or an isolated event, there would be no continuous time. When one perceives a succession of events, there is order and duration implied. Either lengthening or shortening the order and duration of time determines how one perceives the succession of events in the environment. Piaget (1969) has studied time in relation to growth and development in children. Time is related to the child's abilities to use the language, to analyze and synthesize knowledge from the concrete world, and to perceive events as a spatial-temporal continuum.

**Time is unidirectional.** The growth, development, and differentiation in living organisms give evidence of this characteristic of time. Irreversibility is implied in movement that indicates order in life's process. Because life is viewed as a continuous dynamic succession of changes, and there is movement that is ongoing, there is a future element in a concept of time. Time moves from past to the future. As you read these words, these moments in your life can never be replayed. You can return to the above paragraph and reread it, but this rereading will connote a different moment in time than when you initially read it. This moment will never occur again. One element in human beings that differentiates them from other forms of life is this ability to reflect on the past because of information stored in the memory. Have you ever spoken something to another person and wish you could take back the statement? Once spoken the words can never be changed. Another example of time's irreversibility is that lack of sleep during one week can never be made up during the next week as that time is past. This characteristic also identifies time as a continuous flow of events.

**Time is measurable.** Some measurement of time has been implied from primitive human existence by the rising and setting of the sun and the light and dark of the environment. The invention of the clock gave a more precise measurement of time periods based on seconds, minutes, hours, days. The introduction of calendars provided means to measure weeks, months, and years. Human perception of time varies from one person to another and is determined by age, education, position in life, social roles, values, and attitudes.

Studies of changes in body temperature on the perception of time (Orme, 1969, p. 142; Alderson, 1974, p. 42) have shown that a time interval seemed shorter when body temperature rose. Piaget (1969) and Fraisse (1963) explored the difference in time as experienced by child and adult. Adults have learned how to measure units in estimating time. Young children do not begin to develop a concept of time until about 10 years of age. Measurement of time is based on the growth of individuals, and the development of their linguistic and memory abilities. It is possible that metabolic and hormonal processes account for time passing more slowly for elderly adults than for children and young adults.

**Time is subjective.** Time is based on people's perceptions of succession of events in life. Time is relational: successive events follow one another and are related. This succession provides human beings with some constancy in the environment because they can recall past events, relate them to present occurrences, and begin to predict future events. Time is durational and related to movement. For example, when we are happy, time seems to move with great speed; when we are sad, time tends to move slowly. The passage of time varies with one's perception of events. Time is measurable through the use of clocks and calendars. Subjective time helps us measure the probability that having achieved goals in the past, one can expect to use that knowledge to plan to achieve goals in the future. Rhythmicity is integral to a concept of time and is observable and measurable in areas of sleep, day–night cycles, hormonal secretions, metabolic changes, fluctuations in blood pressure, temperature, respirations, pulse rates, and fluid and electrolyte balance. There are exogenous and endogenous factors that influence one's concept of time.

## DEFINITION OF TIME

Time is defined as the duration between the occurrence of one event and the occurrence of another event. It is a change from one state to another state. Time gives unity to large areas of one's experience. Time can only be defined in terms of the observer. Time gives order to the world. One's perception of time relates to those elements that give some constancy in the environment.

Time is a sequence of events moving onward to the future and influenced by the past. Time is a happening, a continuous flow of events in successive order that implies change, a past, and a future. Time is a duration between one event and another as uniquely experienced by each human being; it is the relation of one event to another event. Time is a term used by individuals to give order to events and to determine duration based on perceptions of each person's experiences.

## APPLICATION TO NURSING

When thinking of time in relation to consumers to be served, one might begin with individuals' perceptions of their health in the present situation. Within the hospital organization, time tends to control the many activities of the institution. For example, the day is divided into three time periods, and nurses are assigned to work according to policy each of those three periods at appointed weeks and months. Several studies have indicated the need to pay attention to the rotation of nurses to the various time periods, which are described as days, evenings, and nights, to prevent disturbances in body rhythms (Tooraen, 1972; Smith, 1975; Tom and Lanuza, 1976).

The tasks to be performed for patients in hospitals are allocated specific times of day or night. Medications and treatments are ordered for specific times. Some procedures must be completed in the morning to serve the needs of departments in the hospital. When will the concept of time and the knowledge available about internal body time mechanisms be used to plan schedules and activities to meet the needs of individuals rather than to serve the demands of ancillary services in health care agencies?

Knowledge of a patient's perception of time will help nurses respond appropriately to a situation. For example, a pain medication is requested by a patient; the nurse returns to the patient within 10 minutes after the request to give the pain medication. The patient asks the nurse why she waited 30 minutes to return with it. Waiting makes time seem long. In patients, the alterations in time perspective can distort reality for them. Patients are expected to adjust to the routine of hospitals, to their control of events and independence in decision making that affect their hospitalization. Time is an important dimension in the nurse's assessment of patients, especially those with neurological disturbances.

Sensory deprivation and sensory overload may distort people's time perception. Nurses must be aware of the importance of controlling the patients' environment, if at all possible, to prevent disruptions in circadian rhythms in patients. Examples of the rhythmicity in the functions of human beings can be seen in the body temperature, elimination of waste products, metabolism, fluid and electrolyte balance, sleep and wake cycles, and the nervous system. Changes in work hours from days to nights, some illnesses, allergy to foods, stressors, drugs, and travel are a few things that may interfere with normal body rhythms.

Nurses should assess for altered perception of time intervals in patients. Time perception in individual patients will vary with differences in events and in the situation. For example, it has been shown that increased temperature, pain, and stress will alter time perception in patients. Nurses who have knowledge of time will gather information about time perception and plan care accordingly. Nurses must be aware of those factors in the person's past or in the present situation that may alter his time perception.

Studies in the rhythm found in sleep patterns have implications for planning nursing care to assist the patient to maintain biological rhythms (Fass, 1971; Luce, 1971). For example, in critical care areas, attention is given to maintaining physiological functioning, sometimes to the detriment of other variables such as the sleep patterns. Nurses can plan activities to allow for sleep time. Temperature, pulse, and blood pressure follow circadian patterns. Knowledge of the normal fluctuations of these physiological variables guide nurses in the timing of the measures and the interpretation of the measures. Nurses who assess patients' circadian rhythms can plan activities to enhance their biological rhythms. Nurses can assess their own rhythms and be aware of potential disturbances due to activities required in the job.

Nurses may help patients with their time orientation through the use of clocks and calendars in the environment. Another way to help is through planned interactions with patients in which the patients' time estimation and time orientation are assessed. Smith (1975) indicated that nurses could provide patients with information to help them maintain a time perspective. Nurses should assess patients who dwell on the past and future but deny the illness of the present situation. Nurses interact with these patients and help them set goals and plan for the future.

## Summary

Concepts relevant to personal systems have been presented using one approach to arrive at the characteristics of each concept and then to formulate a definition. Spatial-temporal dimensions of the environment influence perceptions, self, body image, and growth and development. Perception is a major concept because it influences behavior. When human beings enter new or strange environments for the first time, their perceptions of persons, objects, and events influence their actions and reactions in the situation. Personal behavior reflects individuals' perceptions of self and body image. The way in which individuals grow and develop influences their perceptions and vice versa.

This chapter has related selected concepts about dynamic human beings who are in continuous interaction with the environment and whose selected perceptions influence their interactions and their health. If behavior is an outcome of perceptions, then human perceptions become the basic data of human interactions and the facts that nurses must gather and analyze if they are to deliver effective nursing care.

## Bibliography

### PERCEPTION

Alderson, M., Effect of Increased Body Temperature on the Perception of Time, *Nursing Research*, 23(1), January-February 1974, 43-49.

Allport, F. H., *Theories of Perception and the Concept of Structure*, John Wiley & Sons, New York, 1955.

Anderson, M. D., and Pletcha, J. M., Emergency Room Patient's Perceptions Of Stressful Life Events, *Nursing Research*, 23(5), September-October 1974, 378-383.

Ashby, W. R., *Design for a Brain*, John Wiley & Sons, New York, 1960.

Bayer, M., Community Diagnosis through Sight, Sense, and Sound, *Nursing Outlook*, 21(11), November 1973, 712-713.

Bolin, R. H., Sensory Deprivation: An Overview, *Nursing Forum*, 13, 1974, 241-358.

Bruegel, M. A., Relationship of Preoperative Anxiety to Perception of Postoperative Pain, *Nursing Research*, 20(1), February 1971, 26-31.

Bruner, J. S., On Perceptual Readiness, in *Beyond the Information Given*, edited by J. M. Anglin, Norton, New York, 1973, pp. 7-14.

Bruner, J. S., and Krech, W. (eds.), *Perception and Personality*, Greenwood Press, New York, 1968.

Brunswick, E., Representative Design and Probability Theory in a Functional Psychology, *Psychology Review*, 62, 1955, 193-217.

Carterrette, E. C., and Friedman, M. P., *Handbook of Perception*, Academic Press, New York, 1974.

Combs, A. W., and Snygg, D., *Individual Behaviors: A Perceptual Approach to Behavior*, rev. ed., Harper & Row, New York, 1959.

Copp, L., A Projective Cartoon Investigation of Nurse-Patient Psychodramatic Role Perception and Expectation, *Nursing Research*, 20(2), March-April 1971, 100-112.

Davitz, L. J., and Pendleton, S. K., Nurses' Inferences of Suffering, *Nursing Research*, 18(2), March-April 1969, 100-107.

Dawson, N., and Stern, M., Perceptions of Priorities for Home Nursing Care, *Nursing Research*, 22(2), March-April 1973, 145-148.

Dixon, J. K., and Koerner, B., Faculty and Student Perceptions of Effective Classroom Teaching in Nursing, *Nursing Research*, 25(4), July-August 1976, 300-305.

Dodge, J., Factors Related to Patients' Perception of Their Cognitive Needs, *Nursing Research*, 18(6), November-December 1969, 502-512.

Downs, F., Bedrest and Sensory Disturbances, *American Journal of Nursing*, 74(3), March 1974, 434-438.

Ellis, R., Unusual Sensory and Thought Disturbances after Cardiac Surgery, *American Journal of Nursing*, 72(11), November 1972, 2021-2025.

Folta, J. R., The Perception of Death, *Nursing Research*, 14(2), Summer 1965, 232-235.

Forsyth, G. L., Analysis of the Concept of Empathy: Illustration of One Approach, *Advances in Nursing Science*, 2(2), January 1980, 33-42.

Gibson, E. J., *Principles of Perceptual Learning and Development*, Appleton-Century-Crofts, New York, 1969.

Gibson, J., *The Senses Considered as Perceptual Systems,* Houghton Mifflin, Boston, 1966.

Gimbel, L., The Pathology of Boredom and Sensory Deprivation, *Psychiatric Nursing*, 16, September-October 1975, 12-30.

Harrington, H. A., and Theis, E. C., Institutional Factors Perceived by Baccalaureate Students as Influencing Their Performance as Staff Nurses, *Nursing Research*, 17(3), May-June 1968, 228-235.

Hastorf, A. H., Schneider, D. J., and Polefka, J., *Person Perception*, Addison-Wesley, Reading, Massachusetts, 1970.

Ittleson, W., and Cantril, H., *Perception: A Transactional Approach,* Doubleday, Garden City, N.Y., 1954.

Jackson, W. E., and Ellis, R., Sensory Deprivation as a Field of Study, *Nursing Research*, 20(1), January-February 1971, 46-54.

Jarvis, D., Open Heart Surgery: Patients' Perceptions of Care, *American Journal of Nursing*, 70(12), December 1970, 2591-2593.

Joelson, M., and Joelson, R., Do Perceptual Changes Occur in Crisis? A Care Study, *Journal of Psychiatric Nursing*, 10, September-October 1972, 6-10.

Johnson, J., and Rice, V., Sensory and Distress Components of Pain, *Nursing Research*, 23(3), May–June 1974, 203–209.

Johnson, J., Kirchhoff, K., and Endress, M. P., Altering Children's Distress Behavior during Orthopedic Case Removal, *Nursing Research*, 24(6), November–December 1975, 404–410.

Johnson, J. E., Effects of Structuring Patients' Expectations of Their Relation to Threatening Events, *Nursing Research*, 21(6), November–December 1972, 599–604.

Kaufman, M. A., Identification of a Theoretical Basis for Nursing Practice, Ph.D. dissertation, University of California, Los Angeles, 1958.

Kelley, K. J., and Hammond, K. R., An Approach to the Study of Clinical Inference, *Nursing Research*, 13(4), Fall 1964, 314–322.

Kibrick, A. K., Drop Outs in Schools of Nursing: The Effect on Self and Role Perception, *Nursing Research*, 12(3), Summer 1973, 140–149.

King, I. M., A Conceptual Frame of Reference for Nursing, *Nursing Research*, 16(1), January–February 1968, 27–30.

King, I. M., *Toward a Theory for Nursing*, John Wiley & Sons, New York, 1971.

Klein, G., *Perception, Motivation and Personality*, Knopf, New York, 1970.

Laing, R. D., Phillipson, H., and Lee, A. R. *Interpersonal Perception*, Harper & Row, New York, 1966.

Larson, P. A., Influence of Patient Status and Health Condition on Nurse Perceptions of Patient Characteristics, *Nursing Research*, 26(4), July–August 1977, 416–421.

Lewin, K., Field Theory and Learning, in *Field Theory and Social Science*, edited by D. Cartwight, Harper & Row, New York, 1951.

McCaffery, M., Children's Response to Rectal Temperatures: An Exploratory Study, *Nursing Research*, 20(1), January–February 1971, 32–45.

Marriner, A., The Student's Perception of His Creativity, *Nursing Research*, 26(1), January–February 1977, 57.

Merrow, D. L., and Johnson, B. S., Perceptions of the Mother's Role with Her Hospitalized Child, *Nursing Research*, 17(2), March–April 1968, 155–15.

Miller, J., Cognitive Dissonance in Modifying Family Perceptions, *American Journal of Nursing*, 74(8), August 1974, 1468–1470.

Muhlenkamp, A. F., Gress, L. D., and Flood, M. A., Perception of Life Change Events by the Elderly, *Nursing Research*, 24(2), March–April 1975, 109–113.

Mulcahy, R. A., and Janz, N., Effectiveness of Raising Pain Perception Threshold in Males and Females Using a Prophylactic Childbirth Technique during Induced Pain, *Nursing Research*, 22(5), September–October 1973, 423–427.

Murray, R., and Zentner, J. *Nursing Concepts for Health Promotion*, Prentice-Hall, Englewood Cliffs, New Jersey, 1978.

Orlando, I. J., *The Dynamic Nurse–Patient Relationship*, Putnam's, New York, 1961.

Orlando, I. J., *The Discipline and Teaching of Nursing Process*, Putnam's, New York, 1972.

Palmer, I. S., The Development of a Measuring Device: Measuring Patients' Perception toward Impending Surgery, *Nursing Research*, 14(2), Spring 1965, 100–105.

Pearson, B., Use of the Five Senses in Acquiring Professional Skills, *Nursing Research*, 23, May–June 1974, 259–262.

Piaget, J., *The Mechanisms of Perception*, Basic Books, New York, 1969.

Porter, C. S., Grade-School Children's Perceptions of Their Internal Body Parts, *Nursing Research*, 23(5), September–October 1974, 384–391.

Powers, W., *Behavior: The Control of Perception*, Aldine, Chicago, 1973.

Rawlinson, M. R., Projection in Relation to Interpersonal Perception, *Nursing Research*, 14(2), Spring 1965, 114–118.

Schultz, N. V., How Children Perceive Pain, *Nursing Outlook*, 19(10), October 1971, 670–673.

Smolinski, L. M., Patient Perceptions of Care Received and Nurse Perceptions of Care Given Regarding the Same Nursing Acts. Ph.D. dissertation, The Catholic University of American, Washington, D.C., 1975.

Taguiri, R., and Petrullo, L., *Person Perception and Interpersonal Behavior*, Stanford University Press, Stanford, California, 1958.

Thompson, L. R., Sensory Deprivation: A Personal Experience, *American Journal of Nursing*, 73(2), February 1973, 266–268.

Torres, G., Educator's Perceptions of Evolving Nursing Functions, *Nursing Outlook*, 22(3), March 1974, 184–187.

Verhonick, P., et al., I Came, I Saw, I Responded: Nursing Observation and Action Survey, *Nursing Research*, 17(1), January–February 1968, 38–44.

Volicer, B. J., Perceived Stress Levels of Events Associated with the Experience of Hospitalization, *Nursing Research*, 22(6), November–December 1973, 491–497.

Volicer, B. J., Patients Perceptions of Stressful Events Associated with Hospitalization, *Nursing Research*, 23(3), May–June 1974, 235–238.

Weintraub, D., and Walker, E., *Perception*, Brooks/Cole, Belmont, California, 1966.

Whiting, J. F., Q-Sort: A Technique for Evaluating Perceptions of Interpersonal Relationships, *Nursing Research*, 4, October 1955, 70–73.

Whiting, J. F., Patient Needs, Nurses Needs and the Healing Process, *American Journal of Nursing*, 59(5), May 1959, 611–615.

Williamson, Y. M., Methodological Dilemmas in Tapping the Concept of Patient Needs, *Nursing Research*, 27(3), May–June 1978, 172–177.

Wilson, J., *Thinking with Concepts*, Cambridge University Press, London, 1963.

Woods, N., and Falk, S., Noise Stimuli in the Acute Care Area, *Nursing Research*, 23(2), March–April 1974, 144–150.

## SELF AND BODY IMAGE

Blackwell, B., Stigma, in *Behavioral Concepts and Nursing Intervention*, edited by C. E. Carlson, Lippincott, Philadelphia, 1970, pp. 317–327.

Blaesing, S., and Brockhaus, J., The Development of Body Image in the Child, *The Nursing Clinics of North America*, 7(4), December 1972, 598.

Braden, C. J., and Price, J. L., Encouraging Client Self-Discovery, *American Journal of Nursing*, 76(3), March 1976, 444-446.

Buber, M., *I and Thou*, Scribner's, New York, 1970.

Castell, A., *The Self in Philosophy*, Macmillan, New York, 1965.

Cole, P., *The Problematic Self in Kierkegaard and Freud*, Yale University Press, New Haven, 1972.

Colliton, M. (ed.), The Use of Self in Clinical Practice, *The Nursing Clinics of North America*, 6(4), Saunders, Philadelphia, December 1971.

Corbeil, M., Nursing Process for a Patient with a Body Image Disturbance, *The Nursing Clinics of North America*, 6, March 1971, 155-163.

Craft, C., Body Image and Obesity, *The Nursing Clinics of North America*, 7(4), December 1972, 677-685.

Crate, M., Nursing Functions in Adaptation to Chronic Illness, *American Journal of Nursing*, 75(10), October 1975, 72-76.

Dempsey, M., The Development of Body Image in the Adolescent, *The Nursing Clinics of North America*, 7(4), December 1972, 609-615.

Elkin, F., Socialization and the Presentation of Self, in *Family Roles and Interaction: An Anthology*, edited by J. Heiss, 2nd ed., Rand-McNally, Chicago, 1976.

Erikson, E., *Childhood and Society*, Norton, New York, 1963.

Fisher, S., *Body Consciousness: You Are What You Feel*, Prentice-Hall, Englewood Cliffs, New Jersey, 1973.

Fisher, S., and Cleveland, S., *Body Image and Personality*, Dover, New York, 1968.

Gallagher, A., Body Image Changes in the Patient with a Colostomy, *The Nursing Clinics of North America*, 8(4), December 1973, 669-676.

Gergen, J., *The Concept of Self*, Holt, Rinehart & Winston, New York, 1971.

Goffman, E., *The Presentation of Self in Everyday Life*, Doubleday, Garden City, New York, 1959.

Goffman, E., *Stigma*, Prentice-Hall, Englewood Cliffs, New Jersey, 1965.

Gruendemann, B., The Impact of Surgery on Body Image, *The Nursing Clinics of North America*, 10(4), December 1975, 635-642.

Hall, C., and Lindzey, G., *Theories of Personality*, 3rd ed., John Wiley & Sons, New York, 1978.

Hewitt, J. P., *Self and Society: A Symbolic Interactionist in Social Psychology*, Allyn & Bacon, Boston, 1976.

Jersild, A. T., *In Search of Self*, Columbia University, Teachers College Press, New York, 1952.

Jourard, S. M., *The Transparent Self*, Van Nostrand, New York, 1971.

Jung, C., *The Undiscovered Self*, Little, Brown, Boston, 1958.

Kolb, L. C., Disturbances of Body Image, in *American Handbook of Psychiatry*, edited by S. Arieti, Basic Books, New York, 1959, pp. 749-769.

Laing, R. D., *The Divided Self*, Penguin Books, Baltimore, 1965.

Leonard, B., Body Image Changes in Chronic Illness, *The Nursing Clinics of North America*, 7(4), December 1972, 687-695.

Loxley, A., The Emotional Toll of Crippling Deformity, *American Journal of Nursing*, 72(10), October 1972, 1839–1840.

Maier, H. W., *Three Theories of Child Development*, Harper & Row, New York, 1965.

Maltz, M., *Psycho-Cybernetics*, Pocket Books, New York, 1975.

May, R., *Man's Search for Himself*, Norton, New York, 1953.

McCloskey, J., How to Make the Most of Body Image Theory in Nursing Practice, *Nursing 76*, 6(5), May 1976, 68–72.

Murray, R., Body Image Development in Adulthood, *The Nursing Clinics of North America*, 7(4), December 1972, 617–630.

Murray, R., Principles of Nursing Intervention for Adult Patients with Body Image Changes, *The Nursing Clinics of North America*, 7(4), December 1972, 696–707.

Myers, G., *Self: An Introduction to Philosophical Psychology*, Western Publishing, New York, 1969.

Norris, C. M., The Professional Nurse and Body Image, in *Behavioral Concepts and Nursing Intervention*, edited by C. Carlson and B. Blackwell, Lippincott, Philadelphia, 1970, pp. 5–36.

Peplau, H, *Interpersonal Relations in Nursing*, Putnam's, New York, 1952.

Powell, J., *Why Am I Afraid to Tell You Who I Am?* Argus Communications, Niles, Illinois, 1969.

Prather, Hugh, *Notes to Myself*, Real People Press, Provo, Utah, 1970.

Riddle, I., Nursing Intervention to Promote Body Image Integrity in Children, *The Nursing Clinics of North America*, December 1972, 655.

Roberts, S., *Behavioral Concepts and the Critically Ill Patient*, Prentice-Hall, Englewood Cliffs, New Jersey, 1976.

Rogers, C., *On Becoming a Person*, Houghton Mifflin, Boston, 1961.

Schilder, P., *The Image and Appearance of the Human Body*, International Universities Press, New York, 1951.

Shontz, F., *Perceptual and Cognitive Aspects of Body Experience*, Academic Press, New York, 1969.

Smith, C., Body Image Changes after Myocardial Infarction, *The Nursing Clinics of North America*, 7(4), December 1972, 663–668.

Snyder, J. C., and Wilson, M. F., Elements of a Psychological Assessment, *American Journal of Nursing*, 77(2), February 1977, 235–241.

Snygg, D., and Combs, A. W., *Individual Behavior*, Harper & Row, New York, 1949.

Spire, R. H., Photographic Self-Image Confrontation, *American Journal of Nursing*, 73(7), July 1973, 1207–1210.

Timiras, P. S., *Developmental Physiology and Aging*, Macmillan, New York, 1972.

Waechter, E., and Blake, F., *Nursing Care of Children*, Lippincott, Philadelphia, 1976.

Wapner, S., and Werner, H. (eds.), *The Body Percept*, Random House, New York, 1965.

Wells, L. E., and Marvell, G., *Self-Esteem: Its Conceptualization and Measurement*, Sage Publications, Beverly Hills, California, 1976.

Wells, R., Body Image and Surgical Alterations, *Association of Operating Room Nurses Journal*, 21(5), April 1975, 812–815.

# GROWTH AND DEVELOPMENT

Babson, F., Growth and Low Birth Weight Infants, *The Journal of Pediatrics*, 77(1), July 1970, 11-18.

Beck, G., and Vandenberg, B. J., The Relationship of the Rate of Intrauterine Growth to Low Birth Weight Infants' Later Growth, *The Journal of Pediatrics*, 86(4), April 1975, 504-511.

Brazleton, T. B., *Infants and Mothers: Differences in Development*, Delacorte Press, New York, 1969.

Brown, J., and Hepler, R., Stimulation—A Corollary to Physical Care, *American Journal of Nursing*, 76(4), April 1976, 578-581.

Chambers, N., Crawley, R., and Rose, S., *The Biological Basis of Behavior*, Harper & Row, New York, 1971.

Chamorro, I. L., Davis, M. L., Green, D., and Kramer, M., Development of an Instrument to Measure Premature Infant Behavior and Caretaker Activities, *Nursing Research*, 22(4), July-August 1973, 300-309.

Cox, N., Psychological Effects of Surgery on Children, *AORN Journal*, 24, 1976, 426.

Erikson, E., *Childhood and Society*, Norton, New York, 1950.

Forman, R., *Charting Intellectual Development: A Practical Guide to Piagetian Task*, Charles C Thomas, Springfield, Illinois, 1976.

Freud, S. *Introductory lectures on Psychoanalysis,* translated by J. Strachey, Norton, N.Y., 1966.

Gentry, E., and Paris, L. M., Tools to Evaluate Child Development, *American Journal of Nursing*, 67(12), December 1967, 2544-2545.

Gesell, A., *Infant Development*, Harper Bros., New York, 1952.

Havighurst, R., *Human Development and Education*, McKay, New York, 1953.

Helvie, C. O., Factors Predictive of Adolescent Behavior, *Nursing Research Conference*, American Nurses' Association, 6, 1970, 18-64.

Holaday, B. J., Achievement Behavior in Chronically Ill Children, *Nursing Research*, 23(1), January-February 1974, 25-30.

Inhelder, B., and Piaget, J., *The Early Growth of Logic in the Child*, Norton, New York, 1964.

Kaluger, G., and Kaluger, M., *Human Development: The Span of Life*, Mosby, St. Louis, 1974.

Katz, V., Auditory Stimulation and Development Behavior of the Premature Infant, *Nursing Research*, 20(3), May-June 1971, 196-201.

Kramer, M., Chamorro, I., Green, D., and Knudson, F., Extra Tactile Stimulation of the Premature Infant, *Nursing Research*, 24(5), September-October 1975, 324-334.

Krueger, J. M., A Spectrographic Analysis of the Differing Cries of a Normal Two Month Old Infant, *Nursing Research*, 19(5), September-October 1970, 459-463.

MacCarthy, J., and Morison, J., Explanatory Test of a Method of Studying Illness among Preschool Children, *Nursing Research*, 21(4), July-August 1972, 319-326.

Mussen, P., Conger, J., and Kagan, J., *Child Development and Personality*, Harper & Row, New York, 1974.

Neal, M. V., The Relationship between a Regimen of Vestibular Stimulation and Developmental Behavior of the Small Premature Infant, *Nursing Research Conference*, American Nurses' Association, 5, 1969, 43-57.

Neal, M. V., and Nauen, C. M., Ability of Premature Infant to Maintain His Own Body Temperature, *Nursing Research*, 17(5), September-October 1968, 396-402.

Olgas, M., Relationship between Parents' Health Status and Body Image of Their Children, *Nursing Research*, 23(4), July-August 1974, 319-324.

Porter, L. S., Impact of Physical-Physiological Activity on Infants' Growth and Development, *Nursing Research*, 21(3), May-June 1972, 210-219.

Report of the Committee on Maternal and Child Health Research, *Nursing Research*, 26(4), July-August 1977, 308.

Robischon, P., Pica Practice and the Other Hand-Mouth Behavior and Children's Developmental Level, *Nursing Research*, 20(3), May-June 1971, 283.

Smith, J., A Study of the Relationship between Dogmatic and Rigid Attitudes in the Mother and Early Developmental Progress in the Infant, *Nursing Research*, 20(5), September-October 1971, 180-191.

Stone, J., and Church, J., *Childhood and Adolescence*, Random House, New York, 1968.


## SPACE

Allekian, C. I., Intrusions of Territory and Personal Space: An Anxiety Inducing Factor for Hospitalized Persons, An Explanatory Study, *Nursing Research*, 22(3), May-June 1973, 236-241.

Altman, I., *Territorial Behavior in Humans: An Analysis of the Concept*, in *Spacial Behavior of the Older People*, L. Pastalan and D. H. Carson (eds.), University of Michigan Institute of Gerontology, Ann Arbor, 1970, pp. 3-4.

Ardrey, R., *The Territorial Imperative*, Atheneum, New York, 1966.

Bakker, C. B., and Bakker-Rabdau, N. K., *No Trespassing: Explorations in Human Territoriality*, Chandler, San Francisco, 1973.

Barnett, K., A Theoretical Construct of the Concepts of Touch as They Relate to Nursing, *Nursing Research*, 21(3), March-April 1972, 102-110.

Boucher, M. L., Personal Space and Chronicity in the Mental Hospital, *Perspectives of Psychiatric Care*, 9, 1971, 208-219.

Brink, P. J., Role Distance: A Maneuver in Nursing, *Nursing Forum*, 11, June 1974, 47-60.

Davis, A. J., Micro-Ecology: Interactional Dimensions of Space, *Journal of Psychiatric Nursing and Mental Health Sciences*, 10, January-February 1972, 19.

Fast, J., *Body Language*, 2nd ed., Pocket Books, New York, 1971.

Freedman, J. L., *Crowding and Behavior*, Viking, New York, 1975.

Gates, D. M., *Man and His Environment; Climate*, Harper & Row, New York, 1972.

Gioiella, E. C., The Relationships between Slowness of Response, State Anxiety, Social Isolation and Self-Esteem and Preferred Personal Space in the Elderly, *Journal of Gerontological Nursing*, 4(1), January-February 1978, 40-43.

Hall, E., *The Silent Language*, Fawcett, Greenwich, Connecticut, 1959.

Hall, E. T., A System for the Notation of Proxemic Behavior, *American Anthropologist*, 65, 1963, 1003-1026.

Hall, E. T., *Hidden Dimension*, Doubleday, Garden City, New York, 1966.

Johnson, F. L., Response to Territorial Intrusion by Nursing Home Residents, *Advances in Nursing Science*, 1(4), July 1979, 21-34.

Johnson, M. N., Anxiety/Stress and the Effects on Disclosure between Nurses and Patients, *Advances in Nursing Science*, 1(4), July 1979, 1-19.

Levine, M. E., Knock Before Entering Personal Space Bubbles, *Chart*, 65, 1968, 82-84.

Lyman, S., and Scott, M., Territoriality: A Neglected Sociological Dimension, *Social Problems*, 15, 1967, 236-249.

Mehrabian, A., *Silent Messages*, Wadsworth, Belmont, California, 1971.

Mehrabian, A., *Public Places and Private Spaces*, Basic Books, New York, 1976.

Minckley, B. B., Space and Place in Patient Care, *American Journal of Nursing*, 68(3), March 1968, 510-516.

Murray, G., and Abels, P., Domain Conflicts in a Children's Psychiatric Hospital, *Journal of Psychiatric Nursing*, 10(2), March-April 1972, 11-22.

Pastalan, L., and Carson, D. (eds.), *Spatial Behavior of Older People*, University of Michigan Institute of Gerontology, Ann Arbor, 1970.

Pederson, D., and Shears, L. M., A Review of Personal Space Research in the Framework of General System Theory, *Psychological Bulletin*, 80, 1973, 367-388.

Piaget, J., and Inhelder, B., *The Child's Conception of Space*, Norton, New York, 1967.

Pluckhan, M. L., Space: The Silent Language, *Nursing Forum*, 7, 1968, 386-397.

Pluckhan, M. L., Professional Territoriality: A Problem Affecting the Delivery of Health Care, *Nursing Forum*, 11, 1972, 300-310.

Rogers, J. A., Relationship between Sociability and Personal Space Preference at Two Different Times of Day, in *A Source Book of Nursing Research*, edited by F. Downs and M. Newman, Davis, Philadelphia, 1973, pp. 174-180.

Scheflen, A. E., *Human Territories: How We Behave in Space-Time*, Prentice-Hall, Englewood Cliffs, New Jersey, 1976.

Sommer, R., *Personal Space*, Prentice-Hall, Englewood Cliffs, New Jersey, 1969.

Sommer, R., and Becker, F. D., Territorial Defense and the Good Neighbor, in *Nonverbal Communication Readings with Commentary*, edited by S. Weitz, Oxford University Press, New York, 1974, p. 252.

Stillman, M., Territoriality and Personal Space, *American Journal of Nursing*, 78(10), October 1978, 1670-1672.

Suppes, P. (ed.), *Space, Time and Geometry*, Reidel, Boston, 1973.

Trierweiler, R., Personal Space and Its Effects on an Elderly Individual in a Long Term Care Institution, *Journal of Gerontological Nursing*, 4(5), September-October 1978, 21-23.

Watson, O. M., *Proxemic Behavior—A Cross-cultural Study*, Mouton, The Hague, 1970.

## TIME

Alderson, M. J., Effect of Increased Body Temperature on the Perception of Time, *Nursing Research*, 23(1), January–February 1974, 42–49.

Burnside, I. M., Clocks and Calendars, *American Journal of Nursing*, 70(1), January 1970, 119–120.

Doob, L. W., *Patterning of Time*, Yale University Press, New Haven, 1971.

Edlestein, R. R., The Time Factor in Relation to Illness as a Fertile Nursing Research Area: Review of the Literature, *Nursing Research*, 21(1), January–February 1972, 72–76.

Fass, G., Sleep, Drugs, and Dreams, *American Journal of Nursing*, 71(12), December 1971, 2316–2320.

Felton, G., Effects of Time Cycle Change on Blood Pressure and Temperature in Young Women, *Nursing Research*, 19(1), January–February 1970, 48–58.

Fraisee, P., *The Psychology of Time*, Harper & Row, New York, 1963.

Fraser, J. T. (ed.), *The Voices of Time*, Braziller, New York, 1966.

Fraser, J. T., Haber, F. C., and Muller G. H. (eds.), *The Study of Time*, Springer-Verlag, New York, 1972.

Luce, G. G., *Body Time*, Random House, New York, 1971.

Luce, G. G., *Biological Rhythms in Human and Animal Physiology*, Dover, New York, 1971.

Maerloo, J. A. M., *Along the Fourth Dimension*, John Day, New York, 1970.

Newman, M. A., Movement Tempo and the Experience of Time, *Nursing Research*, 25(4), July–August 1976, 273–279.

Nichols, G. A., Time Analysis of Afebrile and Febrile Temperature Readings, *Nursing Research*, 21(5), September–October 1972, 463–464.

Orme, J. E., *Time, Experience and Behavior*, American Elsevier, New York, 1969.

Ornstein, R. E., *On the Experience of Time*, Penguin Books, Baltimore, 1969.

Piaget, J., *The Child's Conception of Time*, Basic Books, New York, 1969.

Priestley, J. B., *Man and Time*, Doubleday, Garden City, New York, 1964.

Sherover, C. M., *The Human Experience of Time: The Development of Its Philosophic Meaning*, New York University Press, New York, 1975.

Smith, M. J., Changes in Judgment of Duration, *Nursing Research*, 24(2), March–April 1975, 93–98.

Stephens, G. J., The Time Factor, *American Journal of Nursing*, 65(5), May 1965, 77–82.

Stone, V., Give the Older Person Time, *American Journal of Nursing*, 69(10), October 1969, 2124–2127.

Tom, C. K., and Lanuza, D. M. (eds.), Symposium on Biological Rhythms, *The Nursing Clinics of North America*, 11(4), December 1976, 569–638.

Tooraen, L. A., Physiological Effects of Shift Rotation on ICU Nurses, *Nursing Research*, 21(5), September–October 1972, 398–405.

van Frassen, B. C., *An Introduction to the Philosophy of Time and Space*, Random House, New York, 1970.

Ward, Ritchie, *The Living Clocks*, Knopf, New York, 1971.

Whitraw, G. J., *The Nature of Time*, Holt, Rinehart & Winston, Chicago, 1972.

Yaker, H., Osmond, H., and Cheek, F. (eds.), *The Future of Time*, Doubleday, Garden City, New York, 1971.

Zwart, P. J., *About Time*, American Elsevier, New York, 1976.

# 3

# Interpersonal Systems

The world is composed of human beings and objects interacting in the environment. In the conceptual framework emphasis is on human beings who function in several types of interpersonal systems. For example, as noted in Chapter 1, two individuals interacting are called dyads; three individuals are called triads and four or more individuals are considered small or large groups. As the number of individuals increases, the complexity of the interactions increases. Several concepts are identified and described that are essential to understanding two or more persons interacting in concrete situations. These concepts are interaction, communication, transaction, role, and stress. Since these concepts provide the basis for a theory derived from interpersonal systems and the conceptual framework, this chapter is more detailed than the others. Since communication provides the raw data for the interactions and for perceptions, this concept is explored and described in greater detail than the other concepts. Common characteristics of each concept are discussed, and the terms are defined. Implications of the use of this knowledge in nursing are presented.

## Concept of Human Interactions

The behavior of individuals has been described as human acts. Human acts are interpreted as actions. Observations of human acts indicate that

59

the perceptions and judgments of individuals are involved in every type of interaction. Since perceptions, judgments, mental actions, and reactions are not directly observable, inferences are made about these components of human behavior. For example, the day before an election the news media and other groups bombard the environment with names and records of candidates. People make decisions about candidates and then go to the polling place, pick up a ballot, and vote. Marking the ballot is called an act. The action is called voting. When people meet with friends the evening of the election to listen to the returns and to the results, they react to the results of the election. For example, if a candidate for whom the people voted wins, their behavior manifests joy and excitement (their reaction). They express satisfaction in having performed the action of voting and in having achieved a goal. The act of taking a temperature and counting a pulse rate is like marking a ballot. The nurse's action is measurement of physiological variables. If a persons' temperature is elevated beyond normal limits, a nurse can observe the person's reactions to this disturbance.

Action is a sequence of behaviors of interacting persons that includes: (1) mental action—recognition of presenting conditions; (2) physical action—initiation of operations or activities related to the condition or situation; and (3) mental action to exert some control over the events and physical action to move to achieve goals. Transactions occur in concrete situations in which human beings are actively participating in the events, and this active participation in movement toward the achieving of a goal brings about change in individuals.

The process of interactions between two or more individuals represents a sequence of verbal and nonverbal behaviors that are goal-directed. Two interacting human beings present a complex set of variables. Each individual in the situation brings personal knowledge, needs, goals, expectations, perceptions, and past experiences that influence the interactions.

A process of human interaction derived from social psychology, perceptions, and interactions is schematically diagramed in Figure 3.1. The diagram shows Jan and Mary, who meet in some situation. In their interactions Jan and Mary are perceiving each other, making judgments about the other, taking some mental action, such as "she can help me with my problem," and reacting to each one's perceptions of the other. Perception, judgment, action, and reaction in the diagram are behaviors that cannot be directly observed. One can only make inferences about these types of behavior. The next step in the process is interaction. Interactions of Mary and Jan can be directly observed, and raw data (no judg-

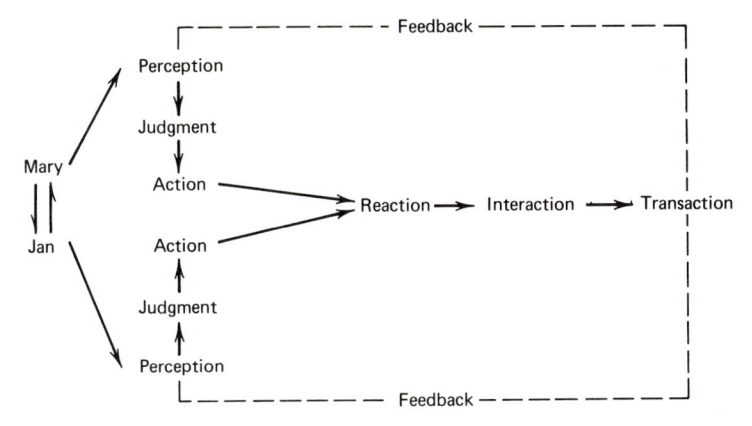

**Figure 3.1** A process of human interaction.

Reprinted with permission from I. M. King, *Toward a Theory for Nursing*, New York, John Wiley & Sons, 1971, p. 92.

ments or inferences) can be recorded. The last term in the diagram, transaction, is defined as achievement of a goal.

The next time you interact with another person, think about this process and test it to judge for yourself. Think about and observe people in your environment who frequently interact and those who seldom interact. Think about the persons with whom you interact. You will discover that either explicitly or implicitly the individuals can help each other achieve their immediate or long-term goals.

In the interactive process, two individuals mutually identify goals and the means to achieve them. When they agree to the means to implement the goals, they move toward transactions. Transactions are defined as goal attainment. The major concepts in human interactions are perception, communication, and transaction. Implicit in the diagram in Figure 3.1 is decision making that is involved in judgment, action, and goal attainment.

A concept of perception is fundamental in all human interactions. Behavior flows from one's perceptions and perceptions influence one's behavior. For example, $B = f(PE)$ behavior is the function of a person interacting with the environment (Lewin, 1951). In addition to perception, which was presented in the previous chapter as a basic concept in understanding a person, two other major concepts are presented as fundamental for understanding human interactions as interpersonal systems.

First, the informational component of interactions can be observed as communication. Second, the valuational component of interactions can be observed as transaction because one obviously values a goal, identifies means to achieve it, and takes action to attain it.

Interactions are a function of individuals living in groups. Hall (1966) identified human activities in cultures, which he labeled *primary message systems*; the first system involves language, while the others are nonlinguistic forms of communication. The primary message system that involves language is interaction. One of the highest forms of interaction is speech.

Communication is the structure of significant signs and symbols that brings order and meaning to human interactions. This structural system includes both verbal and nonverbal behaviors, with nonverbal cues being recognized as more accurate information than verbal pronouncements.

## Concept of Communication

Language's chief function in society is to facilitate cooperation and interaction among individuals. A significant factor in man's cultural growth was the gradual development of language. Language is so much a part of one's daily life that it is taken for granted. Through language persons pass on experiences and thoughts to each succeeding generation. Although words are the symbols of man's thinking, they provide a certain difficulty akin to the difference in perception of reality. Words have different meanings for different people. The experience of the listener, speaker, or reader determines the full effect of the meaning of words.

Communication is an interchange of thoughts and opinions among individuals. Verbal communication is effective when it satisfies basic desires for recognition, participation, and self-realization by direct contact between persons. Nonverbal communication includes gestures, facial expressions, actions, and postures of listening and feeling. Communication is the means whereby social interaction and learning take place. Individuals who are unable to speak with ease, clarity, and assurance and who are unable to listen with comprehension and assimilation may have difficulty with social interactions. To be effective, communication must take place in an atmosphere of mutual respect and desire for understanding. Communication is influenced by the interrelationships of a person's goals, needs, and expectations, and is a means of information exchange in one's environment.

Light, pressure, heat, and chemicals are a few examples of physical energy whereby one receives information from the environment. This information is transmitted through the senses, stored in the memory, and results in patterns of human behavior. Behavior is understood more easily in terms of the processing of information than in terms of the transformation of energy. Communication is an integral part of the processing of information.

Communication is a field of study that is expansive and complex. Multiple studies, reports, and conferences have been published to define, describe, and explain communication. Analysis of the literature shows that this comprehensive concept can be categorized into four areas of inquiry: (1) mathematical theories, (2) theories related to verbal communication, (3) theories related to nonverbal communication, and (4) theories of intrapersonal and interpersonal communication within human beings and communication between human beings and the environment.

## MATHEMATICAL THEORY OF COMMUNICATION

A general system of communication was designed by Shannon and Weaver for the Bell Telephone System (1949). Many people have used their linear model shown in Figure 3.2, and it has been modified to study human communication. This model explains the transmission of information from one source to another. Major elements are clearly defined

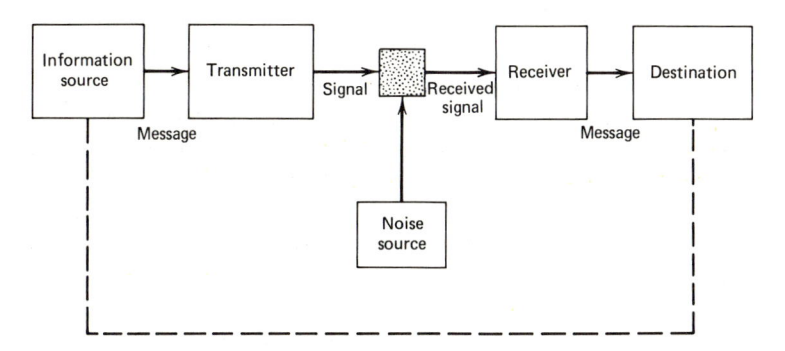

**Figure 3.2**  A general system of communication.

Reprinted with permission from Claude E. Shannon and Warren Weaver, *The Mathematical Theory of Communication,* © 1949 by the University of Illinois Press.

and explained. A feedback loop was added to their original linear model. Ashby and Wiener's work in cybernetics supports the idea of feedback in open systems (Ashby, 1967; Wiener, 1967). Further information about cybernetics and information theory can be learned from works listed in the Bibliography at the end of the chapter. Information transmission is recognized as an essential element in communication. The classic example of the rat and cheese in the maze shows that the ringing of the bell tells the rat to go to a certain place in his space to get the cheese. The bell is part of a patterned environment that gives information to the rat and can be called *information transmission*. When the rat eats the cheese there is *energy transmission*. In human beings, the aroma of food cooking in the kitchen is information transmission. Open systems exhibit specific forms of matter and energy as well as specific patterns of information. Human beings may receive messages (information) that constitute a threat to them. A threat can create strain and stress. Recognition of the meaning of the information as a threat is based on previously stored information about such a message. Generally speaking, all kinds of information are transmitted in the environment; some of the information is received by individuals and some is not received. Noise in the channel (overload of stimuli) by which information is transmitted is one source that may prevent a message from reaching its destination. Another element that may prevent a message from being received is that the intended receiver chooses to ignore the message or the person's perceptual field is narrowed and does not permit the information to be received.

Shannon and Weaver (1949) noted three levels of communication, and called them: (1) *technical*—transmission of information, (2) *semantics*—meaning as interpreted by the receiver, and (3) *effectiveness*—whether or not the meaning conveyed to the receiver led to change in behavior. They classified communication systems into three main categories: (1) *discrete system*, in which message and signal are a sequence of discrete symbols, such as dots, dashes, spaces in sending a telegram, written words in a book; (2) *continuous system*, in which message and signal are both treated as continuous functions, such as the radio or television; and (3) *mixed system*, in which oral speech and music (both discrete and continuous variables) appear. For example, a narrator for a three-day conference may be speaking and at the same time soft music is playing in the background. Schramm (1963) discusses communication, and modifies the Shannon and Weaver feedback systems to include some common experiences of sender and receiver as essential for communication to take

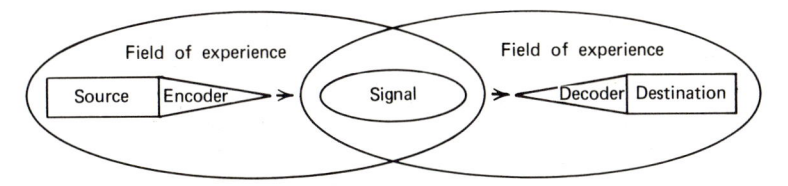

**Figure 3.3**  A model of communication.

Reprinted with permission from Wilbur Schramm, *The Process and Effects of Mass Communication*, © 1954 by the University of Illinois Press.

place. His diagram is shown in Figure 3.3. He explained that the fewer commonalities in the backgrounds of the receiver and the sender, the more difficult the communication. The greater the common experiences of the sender and the receiver, the easier it is for the communication to have the same meaning for the receiver as intended by the sender. Schramm expressed the idea of feedback as an important element in the communication process because it gives the sender some information about the receiver's interpretation of the message. His feedback model is shown in Figure 3.4. In this model, the sender is a receiver and the receiver is a sender. This presents a circular model for understanding the communication process.

A human communication theory proposed by Dance (1967) used a helix model as shown in Figure 3.5. This model expands the concept of

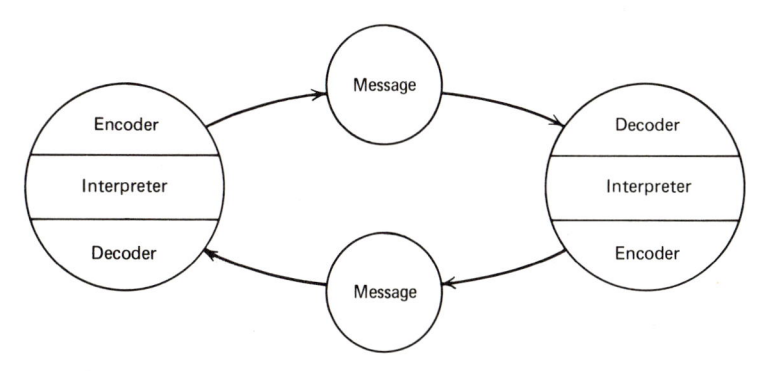

**Figure 3.4**  A circular model of communication.

Reprinted with permission from Wilbur Schramm, *The Process and Effects of Mass Communication*, © 1954 by the University of Illinois Press.

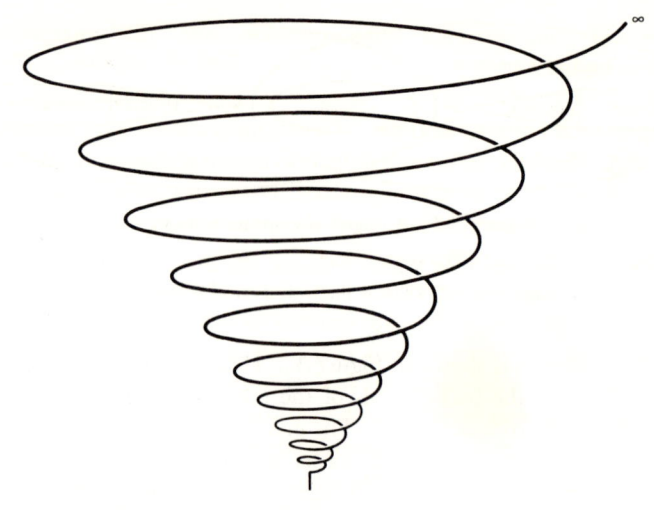

**Figure 3.5** A spiral model of communication.

Reprinted with permission from Frank E. X. Dance (ed.), *Human Communication Theory*, New York, Holt, Rinehart & Winston, 1967, p. 296.

communication to include the idea that past experiences influence human communication and that the model is open, changing, and expanding to infinity.

From these models and the theories described in the writings of the individuals who proposed them, one can deduce some commonalities for understanding the more recent work in the field of interpersonal communication. First, information is sent from one individual to another, the sender and the receiver. This information has been called a *message*. Messages can be sent via a variety of channels, such as teletype, written word, spoken word, vocal sound (a cry), body movements, or gestures. The message may have specific meaning for the person sending it and the same or different meaning for the person receiving it. The meaning is in the person, rather than in the message, although the words or sounds or gestures used may have different meanings for both individuals. The four common elements in communication theories summarized here are language, syntactics, semantics, and channels used.

In open systems, such as human beings interacting with the environment, there is continuous and dynamic communication occurring. For study purposes, these systems are discussed as two interdependent categories: (1) intrapersonal communication and (2) interpersonal communication.

**Intrapersonal communication.** Genetic information is communicated via DNA. Metabolic information involves chemical change in substances from cell to cell. Cells also reproduce. Hormones control the orderly development of human beings, and maintain homeodynamics between internal and external environments.

The nervous system serves as a regulator for human beings and influences communication within and external to individuals. Information is received through sensory neurons, processed, and reactions occur through motor neurons. Any disturbances in the internal communication systems of human beings may interfere with their social functions. These internal disturbances send messages to individuals in the form of elevated temperature and blood pressure, of hearing voices, of thought disturbances, of pain, headaches, and stiff joints. These types of intrapersonal communication are categorized as nonverbal communication.

**Interpersonal communication.** Communication between individuals is classified as both verbal and nonverbal. Verbal is further categorized as vocal, such as the spoken word, and nonvocal, such as the written word. A scream, cry, or grunt are examples of vocal communication, whereas gestures, spatial relationships, and touch are examples of nonvocal communication.

Interpersonal communication is complex and is the information component in all human interactions and interpersonal systems. When one makes systematic observations of a single human being, complexity of a high order is seen. When two human beings come together and interact, the complexity is increased. When three or more individuals interact, one observes complexity of a very high order indeed. Increasing the number of individuals who come together increases the complexity and variability in the situation. This complexity and variability can be observed in large conferences and meetings. When millions of people view the same television program it is called mass communication. Information from whatever source and situation may be stored in people's memories, and influence their behavior at some future time. Interpersonal communication is viewed as face-to-face interaction of two or more individuals.

Several professionals and writers have extended the meaning of interpersonal communication. For example, Watzwalick and his colleagues (1967) noted that communication and behavior are synonymous, that all behavior communicates some kind of message, and that behavior is influenced by communication. He and his coauthors emphasized that syntactics is the information component of communications, that semantics gives meaning to information, and that pragmatics deals with behavioral effects of that information.

Birdwhistell (1970) indicated that individuals are an integral aspect of communication. Communication is not a model of action and reaction. Communication as a system must be comprehended on the transactional level.

Barnland stated that communication is a word that described the process of creating meaning. "Messages may be generated from outside but meanings are generated from within" (Stewart, 1972, p. 45). Berlo agrees that meanings are not transmitted because they are not in the message; meanings are in the person who receives the message and uses it (Berlo, 1960).

Stewart (1972, p. 48) noted principles to be reflected in an overall communication model:

1. Communication is not a thing; it is a process.
2. Communication is not linear; it is circular.
3. Communication is complex and there are six people involved in it:
    a. the person you think you are
    b. the person your partner thinks you are
    c. the person you believe your partner thinks you are
    d. the person your partner thinks he is
    e. the person you think your partner is
    f. the person your partner believes you think he is.
4. Communication is irreversible and unrepeatable.
5. Communication involves the total person.

Watzwalick and his coauthors indicated that communication is the essence of a concept of information exchange. They discussed their concerns that important phenomena have not been a part of the territory conquered by science the past 4 centuries because of emphasis on studying unidirectional cause-effect relations. They noted that important phenomena in concepts of growth and change are influenced by the interrelationship of individual and environment (Watzwalick, Beavin, and Jackson, 1967). For example, feedback is a natural activity in human beings. Self-regulating systems demonstrate that pattern and information are as essential to open systems as were matter and energy to physics at the beginning of the twentieth century.

Cherry defined *communication* as a "dynamic process underlying the existence, growth, change and behavior of all living systems, individual or organization" (Cherry, 1966). Human communication is the vehicle whereby people and organizations relate to environment. Human communication is a flow of information between two human beings through a system of symbols, such as words, gestures, technology. Communication in general means that information is passed from one place to another or from one point to another. To communicate is to establish a common frame of reference between two points. Human communication might be defined as the passing of information from one person to another.

Recent studies have been conducted within a framework of human perception and interpersonal behaviors and in natural settings. Many studies to date have added to one's knowledge of verbal and nonverbal communication. Theories attest to the fact that it is impossible to separate verbal and nonverbal behavior in studying communication (Cherry, 1966; Reusch, 1972; Watzwalick, Beavin, and Jackson, 1967).

The process of communication between two or more persons can be identified by observing the effect of the message on the changing state of the participants. Some of the characteristics of communication can be identified from such observations.

## CHARACTERISTICS OF COMMUNICATION

Open systems, such as man interacting with environment, exhibit permeable boundaries permitting an exchange of matter, energy, and information. Any change or movement of energy and matter organized by information in space and time is action; action is one form of process. Process is the dynamic function of systems and provides for changes in matter, energy, and information. One form of process is communication, which is described as information processing, a change of information from one state to another. Some of the universal characteristics of communication are verbal, nonverbal, situational, perceptual, transactional, and irreversible.

**Verbal communication.** Language provides the symbols that are used in verbal communication. Word symbols have a variety of meaning for individuals. For example, the use of medical terms to transmit information to a nonprofessional may distort the message, whereas, to anyone in the health professions, the words would be clear and have distinct meanings. Abbreviations such as OR, NPO, PRN, and BID have no meaning for most individuals. Words have different meanings in different regions of the United States. In the Midwest, a chocolate milk shake is made with milk, ice cream, and chocolate sauce. In New England, a milk shake does not contain ice cream unless one specifically requests it. Language changes with each generation. Someone may say, *I don't have any wheels*, which means "I don't have an automobile." Someone else might comment, *I don't have any bread*, which means "I don't have any money." Children use the word *tough* to mean "you are all right," but to previous generations it had a negative connotation or could mean "you are a bully." These changes in meaning of words are called etymological shifts. The meaning an individual attaches to verbal symbols influences human interactions.

Verbal communication includes spoken and written language in which information is transmitted from one person to another. Spoken words fly away with the wind; the written word is a permanent record. Speech is one pattern of communication developed in human beings and is one measure of mental development.

One of the first elements in human communication of the verbal type is common language. For communication to have meaning for individuals, one must find a common interest and similar goals. Each person's pattern of verbal communication is influenced by past learning experiences related to language and to situations and events. Listening is an element in communication that requires individuals to participate actively in the verbal exchange. Active participation brings a risk that one's ideas may be challenged. Listening actively helps individuals open their perceptual field to information.

Some barriers in communication may be due to one's inability to listen due to personal or environmental interferences, such as noise or stimuli. Individuals have a tendency to judge a person who is speaking rather than listen to the words used, and they react to the message rather than to the person. If you fear the speaker, such as a person in authority, you may not be able to hear what that person is saying. One's perceptions as well as cultural and age differences influence what is heard. Elements identified as essential in verbal communication are a sender, a message, a receiver, feedback, encoder, decoder, meaning and purpose. These elements have been described in most theories of communication. Emphasis is given to nonverbal communication as a way of gathering information about an individual or group.

**Nonverbal communication.** Many professionals and writers have studied and written about various elements in nonverbal behavior. Mehrabian (1971) noted that over 90 percent of information used in determining people's attitudes or feelings comes from nonverbal behavior and about 7 percent comes from verbal cues. Birdwhistell supported the idea that nonverbal behavior communicates accurate information about another person's attitudes and feelings. He stated "man is a multidimensional being, occasionally he verbalizes" (Birdwhistell, 1970, p. 158). In his cultural analysis of communication Hall (1966) agreed that real feelings are communicated by nonverbal behavior. In his work on touch he observed touch as a receptor of sensations from skin. Writers have indicated that skin is like a cover or an envelope that contains the human being. The sensitivity of the skin places human beings in their temporal–spatial environment. Skin is one of the important media of communication and is referred to by Montagu as the "mother of the senses" (Montagu, 1971). Skin, the protective covering of each human being, is sensitive to cold, heat, pain, and pressure. Skin facilitates a specific kind of nonverbal communication called touch. During the past few years touch has been discussed and studied as an important means of giving information and providing therapy in specific instances (Krieger, 1975).

Touch determines the structure of one's environment and involves the present, a physical closeness to another person as an act of love, an act of violence, an arousal of emotions, a need for comfort, a feeling of presence, or a feeling of pain. Tactile communication influences a person's growth and development. Patterns of communication are established with the way in which a mother holds and touches her newborn. Tactile experiences are learned within the culture in which people are born, grow, and develop. Each person's interpretation of the meaning of sensations received from touch will vary according to his life's experiences within the culture.

Some of the studies in perception are related to touch. Gibson stated that the haptic system, skin, "is the apparatus by which the individual gets information about both the environment and his body" (Gibson, 1966, p. 97).

In observations of mother and infant, bonding and attachment have shown the need for touch. A newborn's life begins with touch at moment of birth. The initial experiences of touch communicate sensations to the baby and determine his feelings of warmth, protection, and security, or lack of these feelings.

Studies have reported that touch is important in the development of children's sense of affection and self-awareness (Mercer, 1966; McCorkle, 1974; Krieger, 1975; Weiss, 1979).

Touch, tactile stimulation, is important for the development of a healthy body image. The feel and the physical appearance of the body is essential in building a healthy concept of self. The skin, which receives the sensations of touch, also serves to protect people. The sense of touch alerts individuals to temperature changes, to pain, to pressure, and to potentially harmful situations.

Human beings use touch to evaluate the quality of an object as to its hardness, softness, smoothness, and roughness. Touch is used in play activities and in learning activities. Touch is a form of communication in some occupations, such as the work of the dentist, the barber, the beautician, the physician, the nurse. Touch has a variety of meanings from one person to another, from one group to another, from one culture to another, and from one situation to another.

A universal characteristic of touch is that it is physical; it involves skin-to-skin contact. What may be considered friendly in one culture, such as two men embracing, may seem inappropriate in another culture. A handshake in one society may mean hello and in another have no meaning. Touch is subjective in that it means different things to different people based on past experiences. Touch is defined simply as skin-to-skin contact of two or more persons. Touch connotes intimacy, which relates to another type of nonverbal communication called distance or position in space.

Distance is a term that indicates individuals wish to initiate communication or to terminate it with another person. People's orientations in space have some cultural variations. For example, Americans tend to stand a short distance from each other when engaged in conversation. Some Europeans tend to move close to the person with whom they wish to speak. Hall has indicated that distance ranges can be described by a change in the tone of voice of Americans. A whisper can be detected when people are very close, 3-6 inches or 8-10 inches. As the distance increases, the full voice can be heard (Hall, 1966, pp. 163-164).

Posture, another form of communication, may be interpreted to mean indifference, inattention, superiority, or concern for another person. Movement of the head when listening to another person speak may indicate that one agrees or disagrees with the speaker. Some body movements are called gestures. Some gesturing with hands, such as clenching the fists, may have meaning in specific situations, where, for example, an angry person shakes his fist at you, or a basketball player throws up both arms with clenched fists as the team wins the game.

Facial expressions communicate a myriad of feelings, attitudes, and information. However, inferences made about facial expressions should be verified with the person if possible. Studies have shown that one should be able to anticipate pain in a patient before it becomes unbearable by observing facial expressions. In some societies joy, anger, frustration, and concern can be detected in facial expressions. Recently, studies have indicated that the dilatation and constriction of the pupils of the human eye give us information about people's feelings. Change in pupil size and reaction has been one observation recorded on individuals suspected of having neurological disturbances. The way an individual looks at another person has meaning that varies from situation to situation, person to person, and culture to culture.

Physical appearance is another form of nonverbal communication. The way individuals dress may indicate the place of business, such as the uniform of a security guard. External clothing may or may not indicate people's status or occupation. Disheveled-looking people with dirty and torn clothes may have had an automobile accident or may not have the material resources to have clean clothing and a place to live. It is not easy to interpret nonverbal behavior from physical appearance without gathering information about individuals in specific situations.

Nonverbal communication sends a message by way of signals or body movements, which mean different things to different persons in different situations. Nonverbal communication is dynamic and in constant change. Gestures are irreversible in that when one gives a sign it cannot be retracted. The whole person is involved in communication and the whole person is responding to the communication of another individual. Nonverbal communication consists of gestures, touch, changes in the pupils of the eye, and a variety of body movements.

A few additional characteristics that describe the concept of communication are mentioned. Communication between human beings is characterized by the dynamic nature of the life space of individuals. For example, change is continuously taking place in each person and in the environment. *Communication is irreversible.* Any verbal pronouncements that are made cannot be withdrawn. Any body movements cannot be wiped away. An individual is never the same person at any moment in time since there is continuous change internal and external to the person.

Communication moves forward in time; once a message has been sent, it is impossible to retract it or know its impact on the recipient of the message. If a parent spanks a child, that spanking will leave its message. The parent cannot withdraw that communication of punishment. This concept has relevance in the health field where it is crucial to have the facts before giving quick responses to patients' questions.

*Communication is personal because each person is different.* When two or more individuals come together, interaction is occurring through verbal and nonverbal communication. The situation influences the context of the communication and whether or not the communication is reciprocal. In addition several purposes are achieved, such as to give information, to reprimand, and to negotiate. One cannot separate self from information that is being communicated in one's environment.

Communication is a process whereby information is given from one person to another either directly in face-to-face meetings or indirectly through telephone, television, or the written word. The multidimensionality of communication can be observed in the continuous changes in cells, organs, and systems at an intrapersonal level and between individuals and groups at an interpersonal level.

Studies in the past have analyzed communication in terms of the source, the message, the receiver without the connecting link, and the process of human interaction with the environment. Findings of these studies have given us bits of information that tend to fragment knowledge about human communication. The content of a message can be inferred, identification of source and receiver noted, and frequency of initiation or reception counted, but this content provides little knowledge about what happens to two or more persons in the process of interaction for a purpose, such as in nursing, learning, teaching, or employer–employee interactions. Some studies have categorized messages as to initiator of requests, statements, content, and orientation. All give statistical data but add little to knowledge of how nurses influence patients in concrete situations and how patients influence nurses through communication. It is important for professionals to understand this complex concept in health care systems. Lack of communication in hospital situations is a major problem. Recently, studies have shown that factors such as purpose, goals, past experiences of individuals, and the context of the situation are a part of the multidimensional aspects of intrapersonal and interpersonal communication. Communicating with oneself through meditation and through relaxation techniques has demonstrated in some instances that people can exert some control over events and situations through an understanding of communication. The energy exchange between providers and consumers of health care has been shown to be therapeutic. Communication between nurses and patients is essential to effective nursing care.

Another factor that makes a concept of communication relevant in health care is the need to document in a systematic way the activities of health professionals so that quality assurance can be identified. Effective and ineffective communication can be observed in the responses and behavioral changes in individuals in nursing situations.

**Implications for nursing.** Nursing care involves knowledge of communication and skills in communicating with a variety of individuals. For example, the manner in which nurses enter the room of a hospitalized adult conveys a message. Nurses who stand at the door of a hospitalized patient give a message that may be perceived by patients that nurses are too busy to come into the room.

When patients exhibit behavior judged to be anger or hostility, knowledge of communication will help professional nurses communicate with patients and try to determine the meaning of their behavior. Usually one finds patients are either fearful, grieving, seeking specific information, or anxious about tests or a surgical procedure. In some instances the patient is actually angry. The important thing is that nurses use communication skills and knowledge to gather accurate information about the behaviors. Experienced nurses with this kind of knowledge know that the behaviors they observe are only a small part of the meaning being communicated.

In recent writings about interpersonal communication, generalizations are made that each person's presentation of self demonstrates communication, i.e., each person's behavior sends messages to other persons in the environment. Some knowledge is available that tells about patterns of communication. For example, one can measure several physiological and psychological parameters of patients to determine increases in stress. These parameters are the catecholamines, increased blood pressure, pulse and respiration, urinalysis, and instruments that measure anxiety.

Nurses are perceived by patients as caring; as too busy to stop to discuss what is happening; as cool and efficient; as disheveled and flighty; as warm, kind, and helping. Knowledge of communication is essential for nurses to give care to the elderly person, to a child who cannot use the language, to an unconscious patient, to an adolescent who is seeking his identity at the same time he has been subjected to immediate trauma from a diving accident, to a newborn baby, to a patient with intractable pain, to the mentally ill person. These are a few examples of situations in which nurses are called upon to use their communication knowledge and skills to help individuals through some interference in their life style.

Another area of the need for knowledge and skills in communication is in interactions with other nurses. Sharing information with a new nurse about research knowledge related to pain or to sleep and its application to nursing requires some communication skill. The orientation and teaching of a new graduate with minimal skills to care for patients requiring knowledgeable and highly skilled care requires communication that helps the new graduate feel secure and capable of performing the functions. Knowledge of one's role is helpful too, but knowledge of communication is essential.

Communication between nurse and physician, nurse and allied professionals, and nurse and family members is essential for safe and effective care of patients. Communication is a vital concept in professional nursing.

Factors that may influence the patterns of communication are the individuals interacting in a specific situation, such as the nurse and the patient. How is the role of each perceived by the other person? What are their expectations of the other person? What are the goals to be achieved in this situation? Are the patient and nurse sharing information so they can arrive at mutual goals to be achieved? What are the barriers, if any, to open and clear communication in the situation? Does the patient feel secure enough to discuss his concerns, his needs, his fears? Does the nurse exhibit an openness in behavior that tells the patient there can be mutual trust?

A patient may ask the nurse: *Do you know when I am being discharged from the hospital?* This question may be interpreted to mean several things. The patient assumes the nurse knows the physician's pattern of behavior. The patient may want to know if the nurse knows something he does not know. He might be asking the day and hour for his discharge. He may be asking what the nurse knows about his prognosis. He may be seeking support from the nurse. He may want to call his family to determine when they can come to get him. He may be pondering the cost of his hospitalization. He may worry about whether or not his boss will replace him if he does not return to work soon. The need for nurses to listen to the verbal cues as well as to observe the nonverbal behaviors is important in helping the patient return to his usual style of life and work.

Another area of concern for nurses is the role they play interpreting messages given to patients by physicians and relevant others. The nurses may be cognizant of the fact that the anxiety level of patients is so high they cannot take in any information. Yet, nurses are bombarding the patient with information and wondering why he cannot understand what they are telling him to do.

It is important to listen and to be silent. Nurses should offer patients opportunities to communicate verbally, but should not force them to do so and should be aware that chatter can be annoying to some patients. Opinions should be withheld unless they have relevance to the situation. Value statements without some explanation may close communication.

The use of clichés (such as *don't worry, you have the best doctor and nurses in the best hospital in the city, everything is just fine, ask your physician, you have to be patient as these things take time*) tend to block communication channels between nurses and patients. Patients know everything is not fine. They know what the physician will say as they have already asked. Patients want someone to talk with them about their concerns. Patients want someone to listen.

The nurse assesses and evaluates the communication between patient and family members and self. For example, a nurse plays an important role in assessing communication between mother and baby. A new mother may be frightened, and this fright is shown in the way she holds the baby. The nurse helps the mother through this period, and explains to the mother what touch means to the baby. The baby cries to have his needs met. A nurse can help a mother listen for the cries; one may be for hunger, one for pain, one for wet diaper; one for attention. Rubin (1968) noted there is a definite pattern of communication through touch between mother and newborn. The mother's perception of the role may influence this pattern. The infant's response in situations where crying stops, baby falls asleep, baby smiles, are all responses to mother's communication.

Touch is important in the care of adults, especially when they have had some disturbance in their speech patterns, such as when they have suffered a stroke. Touch is a means to gather information and a means to give information. Health professionals gather information about the state of a hospitalized patient by applying pressure against an artery to count the pulse. Physicians may palpate the abdomen to rule out any abnormal masses. Attending to the personal hygiene of a patient requires touching through bathing, back rubs, combing hair. Helping a patient in and out of bed and to a comfortable position in bed requires touching the patient. These situations tend to legitmatize touch. On the other hand, patients may refuse to be touched by physicians or nurses. This refusal expresses their feelings and emotions, which give the professionals information about the patients. The situation, therefore, indicates the appropriateness of touch.

Some of the functions of nurses, such as giving injections or performing procedures, require touching. Recently, a nurse has reported and discussed her study of touch as a therapeutic agent (Krieger, 1975). Seminars and workshops are conducted to teach techniques of touch as a therapeutic agent. The relevance of its use depends upon the situation, the persons, the purposes, and the meaning and interpretation it has for those involved.

Touch has been described in various cultures as a way of demonstrating that one person cares about another person. Several nurses have explained the importance of touch with patients with chronic brain syndrome and with aphasic patients (Amacher, 1973; Burnside, 1973).

Touch is used when words seem to have no meaning, such as a squeeze of a hand when the patient cannot talk. When family members are grieving about the death of a loved one, an arm around the shoulder may be a means of showing that the nurse cares. Patients who are isolated need some kind of tactile stimulation. Nurses must help individuals when they are dealing with altered body image or when emotional support is essential to help a person cope with some physical disability. Body image influences one's self-esteem and concept of self, and the patient observes whether or not the nurse stands off from him or shows rejection in facial expressions and body movements. Touch is one kind of nonverbal communication that is essential for development of self-awareness and a concept of self interacting with human beings.

Nurses must become aware of the use of nonverbal communication, its meaning to patients and its purpose. There are many channels of communication and many forms of communication, and each has a time and place and meaning for those involved. For example, when a person is admitted to the hospital for a laryngectomy, it is essential that plans are shared with the patient for ways to communicate postoperatively. It is not always the words one uses but the smile on the face, the tone of voice, the body movements toward or away from a person that clearly communicate a message of caring about the patient and of helping to cope with interferences in health.

Information available to members of the health team is crucial in care, cure, and recovery of patients. It is each professional's responsibility to give accurate information to the other in planning patient care. It is often the nurse's responsibility to decipher the information about patient care to implement plans.

Communication with other personnel in a health care agency is an important part of nursing. It is essential that every department within the agency understands the relevance of clear and accurate information to provide effective care. Scientific knowledge is of little value if one cannot clearly communicate its use in nursing.

Special care areas in hospitals require specific kinds of communication. For example, patients waking up in a recovery room remember nurses who held their hand, smiled, and let them know about the environment. A mutuality exists between the care giver and the recipient of the care.

The nurse must be guided by knowledge of communication in observing patient behavior and in verifying the accuracy of perceptions of that behavior. The nurse has a responsibility to maintain open communication with the patient to mutually set goals to be achieved. Communication between health professionals that is directed toward common goals will facilitate care-giving functions of the nurse.

**Summary.** Communication is the vehicle by which human relations are developed and maintained. A systems approach to communication involves intrapersonal and interpersonal communication in a temporal-spatial environment. Channels that facilitate communication between individuals and their environment are spoken words, written words, gestures, cries, printed books, telegraphs, telephones, computers, transportation systems, and satellites. Understanding communication between individuals and groups requires some understanding of the theories and models that influenced the current emphasis on interpersonal communication.

Human communication is a fundamental social process in that it facilitates ordered functions of human groups and societies. All human activities that link person to person and person to environment are forms of communication. The means used to share information and ideas are verbal and nonverbal signs and symbols by which individuals also express their goals and values. The process of communication expands the world from awareness of self to interactions with others. Communication wears many faces. One source in today's world is listening to the words of others by way of television, telephone, recordings, poetry, speeches, books. In their daily lives, people may experience a variety of communication in fact-to-face situations as well as indirectly. In most person-oriented professions, such as nursing, knowledge and skills in communication are an important part of professional work as communication forms the basis for interactions with individuals who may be experiencing unusual stress that causes them to seek professional assistance.

The relevance of a concept of communication, communication skills, and the value of privileged communication for nursing education is obvious. The ideas have led to one conclusion: all behavior is communication. Communication is the informational component of human interactions. The next question follows: What purpose does this serve for nurse–patient interactions? This question leads to the second major component in human interaction, which is viewed here as achieved goal and is labeled transaction.

## Concept of Transactions

The concept of transactions in the framework presented in this book is derived from theories of cognition and perception and *is not related to the* "transactional analysis" movement. Ideas about transactions go back to 1876 when Clerk Maxwell wrote *Matter and Motion*, and mentioned physical transactions. The ideas of an intimate relationship between self and environment expressed by George Mead (1964) implies transactions of humans with environment. Getzel's organization model outlined a parallel between personal and organizational elements in institutions and implied transactions. Dewey and Bentley outlined three levels of organization and named them self-action, interaction, and transaction. *Self-action* was viewed as "things acting under their own powers" (Dewey and Bentley, 1949, p. 108). *Interaction* was viewed as things balanced against things in a causal relationship. They viewed *transactions* as human beings in action as an integral component of the environment with "extension in time to be as indispensable as extension in space" (p. 123). Their early use of the term implied a systems approach, as they believed that the term *transaction* more adequately described a natural system for man in the world than the term *interaction*.

Dewey and Bentley postulated that humans build an "assumptive world" to carry out meaningful activities to achieve goals. This world is each person's reality, the way each one sees the world, the way each one influences it, and the way it influences the person. These human actions are the result of a transaction in which each person plays an active role (Dewey and Bentley, 1949). When one asks what is the function of perceptions and their relationship to interactions, one may note that accuracy of perception increases effectiveness of one's actions. When one asks "effective action for what?" we cannot understand even the simplest perception without considering the variable of purpose or goal.

Perception is a central concept in studying human interactions that lead to transactions. Patterns of assumptions are developed in one's world of reality and form the basis for actions. Each occasion of life can occur only through an environment, is imbued with some purpose, requires action, and registers the consequence of action. Every action is based upon some awareness or perception, which in turn is determined by the past experiences and present goals.

Ittleson and Cantril noted that the term:

> ... transaction carries the double implication (1) that all parts of the situation enter into it as active participants, and (2) that they owe their very existence as encountered in the situation to this fact of active participation and do not appear as already existing entities merely interacting with each other without affecting their own identity. A situation may be appropriately considered a transaction when it is functionally inappropriate to examine the characteristics of any significant component except for the way in which it is involved in the particular situation. (Ittleson and Cantril, 1954, p. 4)

These authors identified the major characteristics of perception as: (1) *externalization*—facts of perception present themselves through concrete individuals dealing with concrete situations that can be studied only in terms of the transactions where they can be observed; (2) *transactional*— perception never takes place by itself and can be studied only in relation to a situation in which an individual human being functions; (3) *perception as unique*—perception is an activity of each person as participant in a world of events from his unique position and providing him with his own unique world of experience.

The ideas of communication and transaction are expanded by Kuhn. He stated "the question is not whether a particular interaction is a communication or a transaction (it is always both) but whether we are interested in the information or in the values transferred or in both" (Kuhn, 1975, p. 189). He further explained that communication is the transfer of information between two or more individuals. Transaction is the transfer of value between two or more persons. Both kinds of interaction are necessary. It would be difficult to achieve what one values, such as a goal to stay healthy, if information is withheld or is inadequate. Kuhn noted that transactions are an exchange of valued things between two or more individuals. This exchange implies bargaining power, negotiation, and social exchange. Transactions are cooperative when two individuals interact; transactions are reciprocal.

## CHARACTERISTICS OF TRANSACTIONS

**Transactions are unique.** Individuals have their own world of reality based on their unique perceptions. Communication is a component of transaction as a human being communicates on the basis of perceptions with persons and things in the environment. Transactions can be observed in interactions in concrete situations. The variables in the situation will influence transactions. Transactions have a temporal and spatial dimension.

**Transactions are experience.** Experience is a series of events in time. The perceptions that individuals have of their reality is anything that can be experienced in any way under any conditions at any time. Reality is a flow of events in which a principle of differentiation operates. Neither a person nor an object can be described independently of the other as each is a differentiation from the other. Qualitative differences between persons and objects emerge in experience.

A shared frame of reference between two individuals consisting of facts, beliefs, expectancies and preferences provide common knowledge for mutual goal setting. In the course of human experiences, one might search for each person's frame of reference rather than absolute answers to problems. Instead of trying to impose one's values on consumers of health care, one must find a common framework to help individuals cope with life's trials and tribulations.

**Definition of transactions.** Transactions are a process of interaction in which human beings communicate with environment to achieve goals that are valued. Transactions are goal-directed human behaviors. If A has something B wants or needs and $X$ and $Y$ are the variables, then if A gives $X$ to B and B gives $Y$ to A, there is an exchange of either materials or services between A and B. This exchange, which involves interactions, helps each reach goals. Transactions are valued by individuals because the goal is meaningful and is worth achievement. When transactions are made, tension or stress is reduced in a situation.

**Implications for nursing.** All behavior is communication that can be observed directly or indirectly. Experiences can be communicated from one person to another to build a common frame of reference. This can be called a *reciprocally contingent interaction*, which means that the behavior of patients is influenced by the behavior of nurses and vice versa.

Transactions occur within systems of interactions of person with person, person with object, in which continuous motion and energy exchange is organized by information. When there is a disturbance in patterns of transactions, something has disrupted abilities to function, and individuals seek assistance.

In nursing, the unit of analysis in transactions is the dyadic interactions of nurse and patient who come together in a specific place called a nursing situation that is within a larger system called a health care system. Each person's orientation to the system involves professional roles, social roles, organizational roles, and the expectations and perceptions of each person in the situation. In a nursing situation, one person comes for some kind of assistance and the other person, the nurse, is functioning in a professional role with expert knowledge and skills to provide that assistance. Value-orientation patterns of nurse and patient are critical elements in transactions. Transactions as processes of goal attainment in specific situations offer a dynamic area for systematic study of role expectations and role performance of both nurse and patient.

Perception, communication, and transaction are basic concepts that explain interactions between individuals and groups in society. Laing, Phillipson, and Lee noted that when observing an interaction, one must determine if person A is acting on person B's behavior (as A perceives and interprets it), if A is acting on B's experience of A (as A thinks B perceives A's past behavior), or if A is acting on B's experience of B's self (as A thinks B perceived B's past behavior) (Laing, Phillipson, and Lee, 1966). They suggested that a person's behavior is influenced by the perceptions and interpretations one has of the other person in the interaction. They emphasized that the behavior one exhibits is a function of his experience. Value systems of each person in an interaction must be considered in assessing and interpreting behavior.

Psychoanalytic theories and interpersonal relations theories indicated that human perceptions and experiences are key factors in establishing interpersonal relationships. Some of the recent work in perception and interaction has moved these ideas into the realm of transaction (Ittleson and Cantril, 1954; Speigel, 1971; Kuhn, 1975; Thibaut and Kelley, 1978). Transactions offer a unified concept of individuals interacting with environment. Transactions provide the data of human experiences whereby nurses can study holistic care.

Several nurses presented theoretical formulations about interpersonal relations. Peplau (1952) proposed that nurse–patient interactions were goal-directed and that nurses and patients grow in the experience. Travelbee (1971) agreed that there is purpose in nurse–patient interactions and that the purpose should be known to nurses and patients. Orlando (1972) noted that perception is a key factor in understanding nurse–patient relationships as dynamic and purposeful. The author emphasized perception, goals, and interpersonal relations as major concepts in nursing process (King, 1971).

The philosopher Buber (1970) indicated that each person establishes a dialogue and is involved in participation with the other to achieve goals. Buber wrote about self as a whole person, and noted that genuine interaction requires open communication. In the existential approach to human interactions, human beings bring their subjective experiences to the present situation.

Role performance, role expectations, and cognitive processes influence interactions.

## CHARACTERISTICS OF INTERACTIONS

Each human being strives to achieve goals for pleasure and satisfaction. Interactions are, therefore, characterized by values, which influence transactions and goals achieved. Human beings through human interactions establish relationships with others. Interactions are universal. People's perceptions determine behaviors in concrete situations where two individuals come together. Each brings past experiences, present needs, expectations, and goals that influence perceptions in the interactions.

Interactions are reciprocal. When one initiates an interaction with another, an action takes place, each person reacts to the other, and a reciprocal spiral develops in which the individuals continue to interact or withdraw from the situation. Each has something to give to the other that the other wants or needs, which may be facilitated by active participation of both individuals in the situation. There is a mutuality, an interdependence in the situation in which both achieve goals.

In every interaction one can observe verbal and nonverbal communication between two individuals. The way in which each person perceives the communication will determine the response to the other person. Learning takes place when communication is effective.

The concrete situation, the context of the interaction, the closeness of the participants, and the interdependency of each person are factors to be considered in understanding interactions of two or more persons. The experience of any interaction is unique in that the time, place, circumstances, and persons involved can never be repeated. Therefore, interactions are unidirectional, irreversible, dynamic, and have a temporal-spatial dimension.

**Definition of interactions.** Interactions are the acts of two or more persons in mutual presence. Interactions can reveal how one person thinks and feels about another person, how each perceives the other and what the other does to him, what his expectations are of the other, and how each reacts to the actions of the other.

Any human relationship involves at least two persons. Relation implies that persons have a common concern or interest and come together to achieve some purpose. Interactions are observed in time and space as one person fulfills a role that is helpful to another person and vice versa. A person generally reacts to what another person thinks, perceives, feels and acts.

Two human beings collaborate to achieve a common goal. Constructive factors are those that improve collaboration and tend to increase the probability of achieving the goal. Destructive factors are those that hinder the collaboration and that tend to diminish the probability of achieving a goal. The observable behaviors between two individuals are the unit of analysis in human interactions.

**Implications for nursing.** Interactions occur in a variety of situations; in nursing the interactions of concern are between nurse and patient in a nursing situation for a purpose. The primary purpose is to assist the patient in coping with a health problem or concerns about health. When nurse and patient identify goals to be achieved the interactions are focused on goals and a positive interpersonal relationship begins to be established. In nursing situations, it is important to move toward reciprocally contingent interaction where the behavior of one person influences the behavior of the other. To establish this kind of relationship participation is required by both individuals.

One person, the patient, usually comes to a situation in which the other person, the nurse, performs functions called nursing. The initiative to begin to establish an interpersonal relationship rests with the professional nurse whose services are needed in the situation. The interaction process is focused on the needs and welfare of the patient. The nurse identifies the needs of the patient through communication, observation, and interpretation of the information to identify problems and goals. If the nurse has a theoretical basis for nursing, a theory of goal attainment identified in this book is used to gain the participation of the patient in mutual goal setting. This action begins the process of learning more about self by both nurse and patient and about decision making that affects both (but primarily the patient) in helping the patient cope with the presenting condition. Both grow and mature in the process of these interactions. Each brings a self with needs, goals, and expectations to the situation. Working together they experience a new kind of relationship in the health care system, one in which the patient is recognized as having a part in making decisions that affect him now and in the future and is recognized as a person whose participation gives him some independence and control in the situation.

Many nurses have written about nurse–patient relationships as helping relationships (Travelbee, 1971; Peplau, 1952; Ujhely, 1968; Orlando, 1961; Brown and Fowler, 1971). The primary focus of the helping relationship is the person seeking help, the patient, but both individuals are influenced by each other in their interactions that lead to interpersonal relationships. Interpersonal relations are characterized by holism, dynamism, purposefulness, and reciprocality. Interactions help nurses and patients gain cognitive clarity about a shared environment. Interactions in nursing situations can be described as dynamic and irreversible processes.

It is through relationships that human beings establish with others that growth, change, and personal development take place. Effective communication and accuracy in perceptions in situations determine learning and growth of nurses and patients. In most situations, one first views the human being and second the role of each person. Through multiple interactions one tends to view the person as a person. Nurses and patients respond through interactions to the humanness of each other, to the presence of each other, and to the reciprocally contingent relationship. In nurse–patient interactions, concepts of mutually significant experiences, reciprocal process, dynamism, and goal directedness can be identified. When two individuals come together in any situation, the outcome of the exchange depends upon whether the relationship is perceived to be beneficial or harmful. A relationship between two persons indicates how one thinks or feels about the other, how each perceives the other, what they expect, and how they react to each other's behavior.

Factors that influence a relationship are the immediate events in the situation, the needs, the goals, and the expectations that persons bring to the situation, the purpose for the encounter, the roles of the persons, their perceptions, and their ability to communicate and to share information to establish mutual goals. Purposeful interactions require openness in the exchange of information and mutual agreement about the means to achieve identified goals. An attitude of warmth, caring, liking, interest, and respect enhances the interactions.

If nurses are to assess, plan, implement, and evaluate nursing care, a basic knowledge of human interactions is essential. Nurses perform their functions in an interpersonal field. To understand human interactions, nurses must understand perceptions of interacting persons, communication as information, and transactions as values in nursing situations.

Knowledge of human interactions helps nurses gather information from observations and measurement of patients and meet situations with an openness to new information. Physical presence of a nurse is important to a patient. Dialogue is important to a patient. Observation is an essential skill for a nurse to gather information and look for relationships in the events. Verification of perceptions is essential to determine accuracy of the information.

An interaction between two persons, a nurse and a patient, involves a dynamic process that is influenced by the situation. Interactions help nurses gather accurate and relevant information about the patient. Nurses evaluate the patient's readiness for learning, for goal setting, for implementing the means agreed upon to achieve goals.

The nurse and patient meet in a hospital as strangers. With each interaction they learn more about each other. How does the patient view his health state? How does the nurse view it? Are they compatible? What expectations does the nurse have of the patient, what expectations does the patient have of the nurse? What do nurse and patient identify as problems, concerns, and goals to be achieved in the situation? The experience of hospitalization and of illness or potential illness is anxiety producing and requires energy. Because the nurse is the member of the dyad with special kinds of knowledge, it is the nurse's responsibility to observe, measure, verify, interview, and assist the patient. The nurse has a responsibility to search for meaning in the behavior of the patient. It is in using special knowledge and skills that the nurse can help the patient move toward goals. The nurse helps the patient learn more about self and what is happening to interfere with life events. Both help each other increase their coping behavior, and they grow in the process.

A concept of interaction enters into every facet of nursing. Establishing purposeful goal-oriented interactions in nursing situations will enhance the effectiveness of care and produce satisfying outcomes for all concerned.

Openness to the cues in the behavior in each interaction helps each person process information from the other. In the schematic diagram of nurse-patient interactions in Figure 3.1, the term *judgment* is used. In some nursing literature authors have indicated that nurses must be nonjudgmental about patients. It is innate in the human being to make judgments about persons and things in the environment. It is time for nurses to think about the ambiguity in the terms used and to arrive at professional language that is understood by professional nurses. It is necessary to look at the judgments made and to decide if these judgments are accurate or inaccurate on the basis of facts gathered. The term *judgment* as used here means to evaluate a situation and the persons in it and to make decisions based on conclusions drawn from that evaluation.

In the course of interactions, nurses can verify their perceptions. Through interactions, each person gains awareness of self and one's view of others and the situation. In summary, analysis of nurse-patient interactions as dyadic interpersonal systems has identified the essential variables in nursing situations:

1. Geographical place of the transacting systems, such as the hospital
2. Perceptions of nurse and patient
3. Communications of nurse and patient
4. Expectations of nurse and patient
5. Mutual goals of nurse and patient
6. Nurse and patient as a system of interdependent roles in a nursing situation.

Perception is central in human experience. Communication and transaction are essential components in human interactions. The quality of the interactions between nurses and patients may have a positive or negative influence on the promotion of health in any nursing situation.

One approach to the study of transactions in nurse-patient interactions would be to search for: (1) concordance-discordance; (2) satisfaction-dissatisfaction; (3) congruence-incongruence; and (4) accurate perceptions-inaccurate perceptions. Another approach is to search for mutual goal setting through dialogue, bargaining, social exchange, and negotiation. One can measure cognitive and affective growth, and evaluate ability of individuals to cope with health problems, such as living with a chronic disease. Presentation of self and self in role of nurse or role of patient is another area that may be helpful in gaining knowledge and understanding of human interactions and specifically nurse-patient interactions.

The development of a concept of interaction requires knowledge of role since role of one person is defined in relation to the role of another person, such as role of nurse and role of client.

## Concept of Role

Role as a construct is relevant in each of the three dynamic interacting systems of the conceptual framework in this book. A concept of role was placed in this chapter on interpersonal systems because roles identify interactive relationships and modes of communication. They identify self in relation to another and the other in relation to self. A concept of self as an individual is influenced by one's identification with other persons. When someone asks "who are you?" do you respond with "I am a teacher, a nurse, a laboratory technician, a plumber, an engineer"? If so, you are responding in terms of role rather than in terms of self. As persons, we function in a variety of roles. Role is viewed as a relation with another person, a position, and a situation.

The idea of role has been a part of man's history from ancient times through Greek dramas and English literature, when Shakespeare wrote "All the world's a stage, and all the men and women merely players" (*As You Like It*, act 2, scene 7), to the modern day. Anthropologists have written about role since the 1930s. Sociologists and social psychologists, psychiatrists and psychologists have described role from their own perspective of social roles, organizational roles, and role of therapist.

Conway (1978) differentiated between two prevailing theoretical approaches to understanding a concept of role, the functionalist view and the symbolic interactionist view. The functionalist perspective relates use of the term *role* in formal organizations, the symbolic interactionist relates use of the term to two or more persons interacting in any situation. This latter perspective is closely related to a concept of interaction presented in this chapter. However, the functionalist views of role may be related to social systems in the next chapter. Both views have merit depending upon the specific context or situation in which the term *role* is defined and used. The interactionist view of role is basic to understanding individuals in roles in organizations. When role is thought of as a relationship with another person or groups of individuals, it is related to interpersonal systems. When role is considered in social systems it takes on the characteristics of the functionalist view. The interactionist view relates to social interaction. The functionalist view relates to more complex social systems. Role can be considered an essential concept in personal systems (Chapter 2) since the behavior of a person is influenced by a concept of self, which includes one's perceptions, needs, and goals. This aspect of role has been implied in the symbolic interactionist point of view but should be made explicit in the development of a concept of role. The outcome of role socialization is the presentation of self in acquiring a role and in performing a role. The outcome requires a development of interpersonal competence. Knowledge of role and selected role concepts are essential in the education of individuals for professional nursing.

Many studies have been reported that have implications for the nurse role (Mead, 1934; Benne and Bennis, 1959; Bales, 1950). Studies of role in nursing situations have been reported (Malone, Berkowitz, and Klein, 1962; Corwin and Taves, 1962). Johnson and Martin (1958) discussed the primary role of nurses as an expressive one. This expressive role relates to the way nurses function to maintain balance in the system and in individuals. The instrumental role was described as actions that help a group move toward goals. It is this latter role that is prevalent in health care systems today. When reading some of the studies reported in the 1960s one must be cautious about applying the findings to the future. Skipper and Leonard (1965) suggested the nurse role is a combination of expressive and instrumental role as defined by Johnson and Martin (1965, pp. 29-39).

Smith (1965) described components of role and indicated crucial issues, such as the nursing education programs that prepare students to function as self-directed professionals. If the organizations perceive the role of nurses as "obedient servants to the system" or to selected individuals within the system, role stress and strain, if not role conflict, will occur.

Hadley (1967) presented ideas of the nurse role based on her acceptance of the interactionist view of role. She clearly presented one approach that helps nursing delineate its mission. Hadley suggested that the role(s) of the nurse should be defined "in terms of goals and/or sentiments that govern the interaction between nurse and relevant others rather than in terms of the expectations for the behavior of a person occupying the position of nurse or what nurses do" (Hadley, 1967, p. 7).

For example, according to Hadley a primary goal for nursing is "caring for" and "caring about" someone. The primary goal of the organization in which the nurse is employed is coordination of medical and allied professional services. From Hadley's interactionist view goals should be clearly stated and the action to achieve the goals should be separated from but related to goals. In this way, nurses can clearly define their role.

Kramer's study of changes in the nurse's role conception, role deprivation, and role models during the first 6 months of employment as a graduate nurse has had implications for role socialization in nursing (Kramer, 1968). The findings suggested that new graduates' bureaucratic orientation increases with length of employment, that is, the value orientation shifts from an education model of the professional to a work-centered model of the organization. Role deprivation was greater for graduates who retained the teacher's role model than for those who adopted the work-centered models. Subsequent to this study and others reported within the past few years, a movement in nursing to provide experiences for students to learn about the nurse's role and to socialize students into the nursing profession has taken place in undergraduate and graduate programs.

The studies and thinking of Arndt and Laeger about role strain, sources of stress, and role set in nursing administration have provided valuable information for continued study of these concepts in nursing (Arndt and Laeger, 1970). Hardy and Conway (1978) have provided a comprehensive exposition of role concepts and theoretical approaches to the study of roles.

## CHARACTERISTICS OF ROLE

A concept of role requires individuals to communicate with one another and to interact in purposeful ways to achieve goals. In this sense, functions performed in role are dynamic and change from situation to situation. There is an element of reciprocity in a concept of role as a person is a giver in the interactions at some point in time and a taker at other points of time.

There is a relationship between two or more persons functioning in two or more roles. For example, a mother gives resources to a child to help the child grow and develop in a loving environment. The child takes from the mother, but in this giving and taking each participant receives some benefit from the interactions. In nursing, the patient gives information to the nurse and the nurse shares information with the patient, and both receive from the interaction in order to function in their roles. For example, through sharing information in these interactions, they mutually set goals, agree to means to achieve goals, and move toward achieving the goals. Another example is the role of teacher and of learner, whereby both learn from the other, and grow personally and professionally.

Role is learned from functioning in a variety of social systems within a society. Children learn about role in the family; they learn another role as student in school, another role in their friendship group, and yet another role in community activities. As people move into the world of work, they learn the roles of employer and employee.

Role is complex in that the perceptions of individuals who come together in a health care system are varied. For example, Parsons (1951) defined *sick role* as behaviors related to institutionalized expectation systems. He noted that the sick role exempts individuals from performing activities of normal social roles. Illness implies a need for help, and there is an expectation that the person who is ill will accept help. Parsons further explained that illness connotes an obligation to get well; one is obligated to seek help and to cooperate. Often the person in a sick role perceives the health professional as the one who can cure anything, or the one who really cares for and about you, or a friendly visitor, or in some situations as a mother or father surrogate.

Role is situational. For example, one may be employed in role of nurse but perceived as helper, assistant, coworker, coordinator. A patient may view the nurse as the one who cares, who gives information that is helpful, who is a friend. The employer may perceive the nurse as worker who demands good pay and regular working hours, who may not be loyal to the organization, or who is essential to achieving the purpose of the organization. So that, while functioning in one role as professional nurse, one may be perceived in many other roles.

When the position does not specifically define the role of nurse, in which goals for nursing are separate from tasks or activities to achieve nursing goals and distinct from those of other professionals, role conflict in nurses will continue to be a problem in health care systems. Conway's analysis of the difference between the functionalist and interactionist views of role should influence nurses to combine the best elements of both points of view for use in nursing to prevent role conflict. A working definition of role has been derived from the studies and reports on the subject.

## DEFINITIONS OF ROLE

Linton (1936) defined role as a person who occupies a status; role represents the dynamics of status, which is performance of functions. Merton (1967) agreed that, when occupying a particular social status, persons are involved in social relationships, but he calls this role *set*.

Several definitions of role state that it is the behavior that is expected of one who occupies a given position in the family and/or the organization. Benne and Bennis defined role as "a cluster of functions that come to be expected of a given class of workers within positions that they typically occupy in social systems in which they work" (Benne and Bennis, 1959, p. 380). Parsons stated that role is "organized expectations in relation to a particular set of value standards which govern interaction with one or more in the appropriate complementary roles" (Parsons, 1951, p. 39).

Orlando noted that "nursing functions and the principles which guide it when integrated in practice, spell out the role of the professional nurse" (Orlando, 1961, p. 9). Kramer indicated that role is "a set of expectations about how a person in a particular social system should act and how the individual in a reciprocal position should act" (Kramer, 1970, p. 430).

Haas has defined role as a "set of standards and procedures which define rights and obligations of persons in certain social situations, sanctioned by interacting members and authorized by the larger society or particular segments of it" (Haas, 1964, p. 1).

Hardy noted that role has been diversely used. "It has been used to indicate prescriptions, descriptions, evaluations, and actions as well as refer to overt and covert processes, to refer to self, and to refer to other." She stated that "the term is commonly used to refer to both the expected and the actual behaviors associated with a position" (Hardy and Conway, 1978, p. 75).

From these diverse definitions, several elements give meaning to the concept of role: (1) role is a set of behaviors expected when occupying a position in a social system; (2) rules or procedures define rights and obligations in a position in an organization; (3) role is a relationship with one or more individuals interacting in specific situations for a purpose. Role of a nurse can be defined as an interaction between one or more individuals who come to a nursing situation in which nurses perform functions of professional nursing based on knowledge, skills, and values identified as nursing. Nurses use knowledge, skills, and values to identify goals in each situation and to help individuals achieve goals.

## APPLICATIONS OF ROLE TO NURSING

Socialization is a process whereby a person learns values, expected behaviors, rewards, and sanctions so that he can occupy a role in an organization. The role of a professional nurse is learned in the initial educational program and later in the world of work. Some discrepancies between a student's socialization in nursing education programs and the expectations as a nurse in work situations have been identified (Kramer, 1970).

Several role concepts have been defined and discussed with relevance for nursing. They are role taking, role playing, role enactment, role relationships, role expectations, and role conflict.

If nurses are to continue to function in a professional role, that role must be defined by the profession, and the educational programs must provide opportunities for socialization into the profession. Since nurses are primarily an employed group of individuals, the various employers may have different expectations from those of the nurses in the positions for which they were hired. If employer expectations are in opposition to the professionally defined functions, role conflict will exist. This conflict decreases the achievement of effective nursing. Nurses who have knowledge of a concept of role may be able to resolve the conflict in the many events that can occur in positions in health care systems.

An explanation of types of role behaviors expected of nurses will help nurses and others see the complexity of their professional role. The recipients of nursing care have certain expectations of the nurse, such as those of care giver, teacher, friend, and advocate, as part of nurse–patient interactions. There are other types of role expectations related to position in the health care system, such as those of employee, supervisor, coordinator of care. The various allied health professionals have expectations of nurses, in such roles as information gatherer, coordinator of services for the patient, provider of functions when allied professionals are not available.

Knowledge of role is important to professional nurses in order to facilitate their functioning in health care systems. Moreover, the nurse has expectations of self in role of professional.

Interactions between nurses and patients and between nurses and other professionals are goal-oriented and effective when the perceptions of those interacting are accurate. Misunderstanding of role and distortion in perception, for whatever reason, may influence the outcome of care. Understanding a concept of perception is basic to understanding self and the role of professional nurse. Nurses, by virtue of occupying positions of nurses, enact several roles depending upon interactions with relevant others, goals, and activities.

Each role enacted by an individual helps the self shine through for genuine dialogue with another. It is important to recognize when a person is using role to express self and also to conceal self from others. Role conformity is an aspect of role playing that may bring tension and stress. Role conflict in interpersonal systems may increase stress in the environment. An opinion is held that stress has both a positive and negative influence on human interactions. Therefore, a concept of stress was developed as relevant for understanding interpersonal systems.

## Concept of Stress

Asking the question "what is stress?" is like asking the question "what is time?" It is ubiquitous. Stress manifests itself in a variety of ways: physiologically, psychologically, and socially.

At the turn of the century Cannon described stress when he was studying the internal constancy of an organism with changes in external environment. He noted the nervous system's reaction to threat and the "flight or fight" syndrome (Cannon, 1963). In the 1940s a number of studies reported findings about stress. Wolf (1955) viewed stress as a "protective reaction pattern" when observing the interaction of human beings with "noxious" stimuli. At this same time, Schrodinger (1950) expanded on the previous work and described a dynamic state of the "whole organism."

Seyle's original report of his work emphasized biological stress (Seyle, 1956). In his early writings, Seyle identified a "general adaptation syndrome" in which he recognized that the person under stress responds with a unified defense mechanism. As stressors continue to bombard a person, some localization may become apparent, such as in tense situations followed by a headache. He believed that illness arises from stress. In his later speeches about stress, he recognized the whole person's interaction with the environment.

Stress has been studied from a psychological framework. Lazarus identified a person's reaction to stress as a cognitive process in that demands are made on the person that may pose a threat or that exceed the person's ability to cope with events. Anxiety, depression, and stress interfere with a person's ability to respond to and maintain some control over a situation. Undue stress decreases one's perceptual field, which decreases the information one senses and the ability to cope with events. On the other hand, stress sometimes mobilizes a person's resources to react in a situation. Lazarus summarized the field of stress in his most recent definition. He and Monat noted "the arena that the stress area refers to consists of any event in which environmental demands, internal demands, or both, tax or exceed the adaptive resources of an individual, social system, or tissue system" (Monat and Lazarus, 1977, p. 3).

Janis (1958) identified psychological trauma, fear, threat, shame, and guilt as factors that act as stressors in some people. He recognized that stressors of a psychological nature may influence the development of physiological stress and vice versa. Researchers have shown a relationship between the internal and external milieu in a person's response to stressors and ability to cope with events. One conclusion from the many studies of stress from different perspectives is that stress is everywhere and is viewed as a dynamic state of individuals interacting with their environment. Stress is not seen as primarily a destructive force in human life, but is viewed as essential for growth and for building coping strategies. Perception is an important factor in the way a person attaches meaning to events as harmful or pleasant, as satisfying or dissatisfying. Holmes and Rahe (1967) developed an instrument that is useful in studying life changes. Life changes may be the cause of undue stress. Dohrenwend's study of life changes indicated that stress and the likelihood of increase in illness were identified with life changes (Dohrenwend and Dohrenwend, 1974).

Studies by nurses have identified some of the stressors in hospitalization, illness, and the work environment. Several studies propose ways in which nurses can identify stress and provide nursing care that helps patients cope with the stress of illness (Pride, 1968; Foster, 1974). Schmitt and Wooldridge (1973) found that patients who were given information, who partcipated in planned teaching preoperatively, and who expressed their feelings about the surgery were able to decrease the tension.

Several studies were reported showing that a Subjective Stress Scale was useful in identifying patients' stress (Parisen, Rich, and Jackson, 1969). A Hospital Stress Rating Scale from Holmes and Rahe was used to study patients' perceptions of stress associated with their hospitalization (Volicer, 1973, 1974, 1975).

Bell (1977) used the Holmes and Rahe tool to study coping methods and behaviors of individuals who are ill and well.

A few studies have been conducted to determine the stress of the environment on nurses. Tooraen investigated the physiological effect of shift rotation on ICU nurses (Tooraen, 1972). The small sample of nine nurses in four intensive care units in two hospitals does not permit generalization of findings. However, similar studies in other occupational fields have shown that shift rotation and tense environments change people's circadian rhythms, which cause fatigue and reduce worker efficiency.

Some studies of the work environment of intensive care nurses identified stressors in such situations as repetitive exposure to death and dying, which may be potentially stressful due to loss or perceived personal failure. The immediacy of the work to be done often promotes problems in communication between nurses, families, and physicians, and support systems are absent in these environments. The initiation of mutual support groups has brought about some reduction of stress. Aiken and others have noted that patients respond to relaxation techniques, which help to reduce stress (Aiken, 1972).

In some of these studies, stress has been observed and measured from many perspectives: physiological, psychological, social, and environmental. There is some evidence that one needs to be able to identify the stressors that interfere with functions or that change the environment. If it is not possible to eliminate stressors, then support systems should be provided in stressful work situations. Information about impending events may reduce the tension due to the unknown. Relaxation techniques have been shown to be helpful in reducing tension. Stress is neither biological, emotional, or social, but is more than these isolated elements. It is the whole person interacting with the environment where one places artificial boundaries around a segment of that wholeness for the purpose of studying events in open systems.

## CHARACTERISTICS OF STRESS

Stress seems to be an essential component of life. In this sense, it is universal. Stress is not limited by time or place. It is observed in plants, animals, and human beings. It is evident when the weight of a building collapses due to weak structure or when the asphalt driveway cracks from the salt on the snow and ice. Stress is everywhere. The stressors identified in studies indicated that stress requires energy to perform daily activities, to react to threat or harmful stimuli. Stressors have been categorized as physical, environmental, chemical, physiological, emotional, and social.

**Stress is dynamic.** Open systems are in continuous change and characterized by energy exchange within and external to human beings. Events in life may be perceived as pleasant or unpleasant, and these perceptions influence a person's response to them. As perceptions and conditions change so does the intensity of the stressors.

**Stress has a temporal-spatial dimension.** Measurements of life events that show increase in stress are potential predictors of subsequent illness or disease. Crisis in a person's life occurs at a specific time and in a particular situation. As an individual moves from one crisis to another there tends to be an added dimension to stress that may increase a person's stress due to past experiences or may decrease stress from having learned to cope with past events.

**Stress is individual, personal, and subjective.** People respond to life events based on their unique perceptions and their interpretation of the events. For example, a person may respond to a crisis by crying, by withdrawing, by fighting, or by denying it. A person's response to stress is influenced by the stressors, the situation, the time of the event, and the meaning it has for the person. Age, sex, environmental background, personality, cognition, and motivation are a few of the factors identified in research that influence people's reaction to stressors. The increase and decrease in stress is dependent on the way individuals perceive it. For example, a person who has given his first public speech to a professional group usually manifests some stress through dry mouth, moist hands, shaky knees. After several public speeches these manifestations tend to decrease or go away as the person feels comfortable in that kind of situation. From this multidimensional concept, many professionals and writers have attempted to define stress from their own orientation to the term.

## DEFINITIONS OF STRESS

Stress is an energy factor in open systems that is increased and decreased by stressors in man-environment interactions. From the many definitions of stress suggested in the literature, *stress is a dynamic state whereby a human being interacts with the environment to maintain balance for growth, development, and performance, which involves an exchange of energy and information between the person and the environment for regulation and control of stressors.* Stress is the energy response of an individual to persons, objects, and events called stressors. Stress is negative and positive; it is constructive and destructive. It helps people reach the highest level of achievement and at the same time continuously wears them down.

## IMPLICATIONS FOR NURSING

The majority of practicing nurses work in hospitals. Hospitals provide a service for individuals for treatment of illness and disease that cannot be performed at home or in an office. Nurses are continuously confronted by stressors in each situation. The environment of the hospital and special care units are stressful for patients and nurses. The working hours for nurses are stressors if the nurses' biological rhythms are disturbed. Nurses are confronted with death and dying in hospitals, and this is a stressful event. Fears, anxiety, survival, loss, and change in life style are some of the factors that act as stressors in hospitals.

Nurses are expected to decrease stressors in the hospital for patients and families, yet few support systems are offered to reduce stressors for nurses. Several strategies can be used by nurses to prevent undue stress for patients and families. Nurses can begin with interpersonal communication by giving information that is appropriate in the situation, by assessing any disturbance in physiological variables. Patients who have a loss of a body part or a change in body image need help to cope with these stressors. Nurses help patients verbalize their concerns and their expectations by discussing past experiences, by helping patients set immediate and long-range goals, and by offering options for achieving those goals. Giving patients some control over what happens in a hospital situation by helping them participate in decisions that affect them will reduce stress in situations.

Nurses help patients cope with the stressors at a time in their lives when they seek professional assistance. Knowledge of a concept of stress helps nurses become sensitive to the stressors in nursing situations and to use stress in a constructive manner to achieve goals.

Some of the findings from the studies of stress in nursing should be disseminated to practitioners. Some of the assessment tools to measure stressors and manifestations of stress in human beings should be used in nursing situations to provide accurate information about what is happening to patients. For example, when a nurse identifies procedures performed on patients in some intensive care units that prevent patients having sufficient time to sleep, the environmental stress is assessed and activities are planned to provide adequate time for sleep to alleviate some of the stress for the patient. When nurses assess that patients have been in an environment with little or no sensory stimulation, they can assess, whether or not this situation is stressful for patients. Providing sensory experiences can reduce the stress.

Individuals who are hospitalized for surgical treatment exhibit behaviors of fear and anxiety because they perceive the treatment as threatening. Information about the events surrounding the treatment helps to reduce fear of the unknown, and stress is decreased.

Stress is important in daily living and in work situations, in play and recreation. Competitive sports are stressful. Technology increases stress in societies.

Behaviors that manifest stress are useful in assessment of stress level in people. Although it is not easy to identify one or two variables and make inferences about the cause of stress, knowledge of some of the behaviors that indicate increased stress is helpful in planning appropriate nursing care.

Some behavioral manifestations of stress can be categorized as:

1. Exaggerated patterns of behavior, such as incessant pacing back and forth
2. Specific changes in activity patterns, such as when an active person who exercises and engages in recreational activities rapidly changes into a passive person who stays home and sits in a chair
3. Specific alterations in activities of daily living, such as change in nutrition from a hearty appetite to a starvation diet or change in elimination from normal to increase in frequency and amount
4. Changes in perceptions of reality and social interactions
5. Changes in work habits, such as when a person who is on time and seems happy to go to work changes into one who is late and is constantly complaining about the work.

Environmental stressors that should be assessed by nurses are sensory deprivation, such as the patient in isolation from the usual environment, and sensory stimulation, such as too much noise in the system or an overload in the information given to the patient. Many health care workers enter patients' rooms and do things to them without an adequate explanation. Change in the time schedules of nurses and other hospital personnel from day to day prevents patients from having a person with whom they can relate on a consistent basis and from whom to seek information and help. One approach to this situational stressor is primary nursing.

Some of the means used to reduce stress in nursing situations have been mentioned: (1) talk with each patient; (2) listen to each patient; (3) observe behavioral cues of each patient; (4) give adequate explanation of tests, procedures, and treatments; (5) help each patient to ask questions about what is happening; (6) help each patient understand events occurring in the hospital; (7) anticipate the patient's concerns from an accurate data base, and from use of interview skills to gather information; (8) offer each patient options about care, such as whether to shower in morning or evening and food preferences; (9) interact with each patient to develop mutual goals to be achieved; (10) involve family members in the care of each patient; (11) help each patient identify expectations of self and others; and (12) plan for realistic achievement of goals identified.

The situation, persons involved, past experiences, present disturbances, and one's ability to cope with stressors are factors to be considered in health care systems by nurses who believe that one of their responsibilities is to provide care in an environment that is conducive to human functions and to wellness.

One concrete example of the health care system and health professionals creating stress in a patient explains why physicians and nurses must be alert to the fact that their behavior may cause the stress. A 40-year-old woman was admitted to the hospital in acute abdominal distress. One of the young physicians gathered information from the history and performed a physical examination. The woman said she had had diabetes for the past 15 years and has no problems with this disease since her insulin and diet had been satisfactorily regulated. After the physician left her room, he wrote some orders on the chart, and one was for insulin. When the nurse brought the insulin to the room to give it to the patient, she asked what kind it was as she had never taken insulin at that time of day. The nurse told her and the patient refused it. The nurse asked her to explain how she had managed this disease all these years. The patient told her the kind and amount of insulin and the time of day. The nurse told the patient she would record this information and call the physician to change the order. This incident increased the patient's stress and her pain increased. Her comment was "I don't need care for my diabetes, please do something about the pain." The nurse alleviated the patient's stress by communicating the problem to the physician who changed the insulin as the patient had requested.

Volicer's findings in how patients perceive stress in hospitals indicated there is a direct relationship between stress perceived by patients and behaviors of hospital staff, such as inadequate explanation of treatment, diagnosis, prognosis, and unconcerned attitudes (Volicer, 1973, p. 497). If hospital staff are perceived as stressors for patients, nurses and physicians should begin to use findings from research to change behaviors to reduce or eliminate human stressors.

Nurses are in a position to observe for patterns of behavioral responses to stressors and stressful events. Once identified they are in a position to take some action to decrease, reduce, or eliminate some factors that produce stress for patients. Nurses need to use more objective methods for measuring stress in patient care situations.

Stress may be viewed as a factor that is related to a total person interacting with a total environment to perform the functions that bring some satisfaction to daily living. Achievement of goals comes about from human interactions of individuals in social systems within a given culture.

## Summary

Life's experiences are made up of multiple human interactions. Concepts have been selected and developed as substantive knowledge about interpersonal systems, with emphasis on dyadic interactions.

A construct of interaction described human acts related to human actions. Although perception, communication, and transaction are developed as concepts, they are some of the defining characteristics of interactions. All events in life have an element of stress or tension. Stress is a concept that is essential to an understanding of human interactions, and is developed in this chapter. Role is an essential concept to an understanding of nurse–client interactions.

The concepts developed in this chapter and in Chapter 2 provide a basis for formulating a theory of goal attainment in nursing situations. Since nursing situations are primarily located within health care systems, selected concepts within social systems are presented in the next chapter.

## Bibliography

### HUMAN INTERACTIONS

Aiken, L., and Aiken, J. L., A Systematic Approach to the Evaluation of Interpersonal Relationships, *American Journal of Nursing*, 73(5), May 1973, 863–867.

Altman, I., and Taylor, D. A., *Social Penetration: The Development of Interpersonal Relationships*, Holt, Rinehart & Winston, N.Y., 1973.

Bales, R. E., *Interaction Process Analysis*, Addison-Wesley, Cambridge, Massachusetts, 1950.

Barnett, K., A Theoretical Construct of the Concept of Touch as It Relates to Nursing, *Nursing Research*, 21(2), March–April 1973, 102–108.

Barnlund, D., *Interpersonal Communication*, Houghton Mifflin, Boston, 1966.

Bennis, W., Schein, E., Steele, F., and Berlew, D. (eds.), *Interpersonal Dynamics: Essays and Readings on Human Interaction*, Dorsey Press, Illinois, 1968.

Brown, M., and Flwler, G., *Psychodynamic Nursing*, Saunders, Philadelphia, 1971.

Buber, M., *I and Thou*, Scribner's, New York, 1970.

Cantril, H., *The Pattern of Human Concerns*, Rutgers University Press, New Brunswick, New Jersey, 1965.

Daubenmire, J. J., and King, I. M., Nursing Process Models: A Systems Approach, *Nursing Outlook*, 21(8), August 1973, 512–517.

Eggert, L. L., Challenge Exam in Interpersonal Skills, *Nursing Outlook*, 23(11) November 1975, 707–710.

Forsyth, G. L., Exploration of Empathy in Nurse–Client Interaction, *Advances in Nursing Science*, 1(2), January 1979, 53–61.

Goffman, E., *Interaction Ritual*, Doubleday, Garden City, New York, 1967.

Guzzatta, C. E., Relationship between Stress and Learning, *Advances in Nursing Science*, 1(4), July 1979, 35–49.

Hall, E. T., *The Hidden Dimension*, Doubleday, Garden City, New York, 1966.

Hargreaves, W., and Runyon, N., Patterns of Psychiatric Nursing: Role Differences in Nurse–Patient Interaction, *Nursing Research*, 18(4), July–August 1969.

Heider, F., *The Psychology of Interpersonal Relations*, John Wiley & Sons, New York, 1958.

Jones, E. E., and Thibaut, J. W., Interaction Goals as Bases of Inference in Interpersonal Perception, in *Person Perception and Interpersonal Behavior*, edited by R. Tagiuri and L. Petrullo, Stanford University Press, Palo Alto, California, 1958, 151–178.

Jourard, S. M., *The Transparent Self*, Van Nostrand, New York, 1971.

Kelley, J. H., and Thibaut, J. W., *Interpersonal Relations: A Theory of Interdependence*, John Wiley & Sons, New York, 1978.

King, I. M., *Toward a Theory of Nursing*, John Wiley & Sons, New York, 1971.

King, I. M., The Health Care System: Nursing Intervention Subsystem, in *Health Research: The Systems Approach*, edited by H. Werley, et al., Springer, New York, 1976, 51–60.

Laing, R. D., Phillipson, H., and Lee, A. R., *Interpersonal Perception*, Harper & Row, New York, 1966.

Loomis, M., and Horsley, J. A., *Interpersonal Change: A Behavioral Approach to Nursing Practice*, McGraw-Hill, New York, 1974.

Lum, J., Interaction Patterns of Nursing Personnel, *Nursing Research*, 19(4), July–August 1970, 324–330.

McCrosky, J. D., Larson, C. E., and Knapp, M. L., *An Introduction to Interpersonal Communication*, Prentice-Hall, Englewood Cliffs, New Jersey, 1971.

Morimoto, F., Favoritism in Personal-Patient Interaction, *Nursing Research*, 4, February 1955, 102-112.

Moss, F. T., and Meyer, B., The Effects of Nursing Interaction upon Pain Relief in Patients, *Nursing Research*, 15, Fall 1966, 303-306.

Orlando, I. J., *The Dynamic Nurse-Patient Relationship*, Putnam's, New York, 1961.

Peplau, H., *Interpersonal Relations in Nursing*, Putnam's, New York, 1952.

Popiel, E., and Welch, C., Interpersonal Factors as Correlates of Interpersonal Awareness in Training Groups, *Nursing Research*, 20(2), March-April 1971, 165-167.

Rogers, C. R., Interpersonal Relationships: U.S.A. 2000, *Journal of Applied Behavioral Science*, 4(3), 1968, 265-280.

Ryden, M., The Predictive Value of a Clinical Examination of Interpersonal Relationship Skills, *Journal of Nursing Education*, 16(5), May 1977, 27-31.

Tagiuri, R., and Petrullo, L. (eds.), *Person Perception and Interpersonal Behavior*, Stanford University Press, Palo Alto, California, 1958.

Travelbee, J., *Interpersonal Aspects of Nursing*, Davis, Philadelphia, 1971.

Ujhely, G., *Determinants of the Nurse-Patient Relationship*, Springer, New York, 1968.

Veninga, R., Communications: A Patient's Eye View, *American Journal of Nursing*, 73(2), February 1973, 320-322.

Whiting, J. F., Q-Sort Technique for Evaluating Perceptions of Interpersonal Relationships, *Nursing Research*, 4, October 1955, 71-73.

Whiting, J. F., Patients' Needs, Nurses' Needs and the Healing Process, *American Journal of Nursing*, 59(5), May 1959, 661-665.

## COMMUNICATION

Aguilera, D., Relations between Physical Contact and Verbal Interaction between Nurses and Patients, *Journal of Psychiatric Nursing*, 5, January-February 1967, 5-20.

Amacher, N. J., Touch Is a Way of Caring, *American Journal of Nursing*, 73(5), May 1973, 852-854.

Ashby, W., Ross, *An Introduction to Cybernetics*, John Wiley & Sons, New York, 1966.

Baer, E., Davitz, L., and Lieb, R., Inferences of Physical Pain and Psychological Distress in Relation to Verbal and Nonverbal Patient Communication, *Nursing Research*, 19(5), September-October 1970, 388-392.

Barnett, K., A Theoretical Construct of the Concepts of Touch as They Relate to Nursing, *Nursing Research*, 21(3), March-April 1972, 102-110.

Bender, R. E., Communicating with the Deaf, *American Journal of Nursing*, 56(4), April 1966, 757-760.

Berelson, B., *Content Analysis in Communication Research*, Free Press, New York, 1952.

Berlo, D., *The Process of Communication*, Holt, Rinehart & Winston, New York, 1960.

Birdwhistell, R., *Kinesics and Context*, University of Pennsylvania Press, Philadelphia, 1970.

Boguslowski, M., The Use of Therapeutic Touch in Nursing, *The Journal of Continuing Education in Nursing*, 10, 1979, 9-15.

Bower, T. G., *A Primer of Infant Development*, Freeman, San Francisco, 1977.

Brown, M., and Fowler, G., *Psychodynamic Nursing*, Saunders, Philadelphia, 1971.

Buhler, C., *The First Year of Life*, Arno Press, New York, 1975.

Burnside, I., Touching Is Talking, *American Journal of Nursing*, 73(12), December 1973, 2060-2063.

Burnside, I. M., Ebersole, P., and Monea, H. B., *Psychosocial Caring throughout the Life Span*, McGraw-Hill, New York, 1979.

Cannon, R., The Development of Maternal Touch during Early Mother-Infant Interaction, *Journal of Obstetrics and Gynecology*, March-April 1977, 18-32.

Cartwright, D., and Zander, A. (eds.), *Group Dynamics: Research and Theory*, Harper & Row, New York, 1968.

Cherry, C., *On Human Communication*, MIT Press, Cambridge, Massachusetts, 1966.

Clark, A., and Alfonso, D., Infant Behavior and Maternal Attachment: Two Sides to the Coin, *The American Journal of Maternal Child Nursing*, March-April 1976, 94-99.

Cooper, J., Actions Really Do Speak Louder than Words, *Nursing*, 79(9), 1979, 113-118.

Crayter, J., Talking with Patients Who Have Cancer, *American Journal of Nursing*, 69(4), April 1969, 747-750.

Dance, F. E. X., *Human Communication Theory*, Holt, Rinehart & Winston, New York, 1967.

Danzinger, K., *Interpersonal Communication*, Pergamon Press, New York, 1976.

Daubenmire, M. J., Searles, S. S., and Ashton, C. A., A Methodologic Framework to Study Nurse-Patient Communication, *Nursing Research*, 27(5), September-October 1978, 304-310.

Fast, J., *Body Language*, Pocket Books, New York, 1971.

Fox, M., Talking with Patients Who Can't Answer, *American Journal of Nursing*, 71(6), June 1971, 1146-1149.

Gibson, J., *The Senses Reconsidered as Perceptual Systems*, Houghton Mifflin, Boston, 1966.

Haggerty, V. C., Listening: An Experiment in Nursing, *Nursing Forum*, 10, 1971, 383-391.

Hall, E. T., *The Silent Language*, Fawcett, Greenwich, Conneucticut, 1959.

Hall, E. T., *The Hidden Dimension*, Doubleday, Garden City, New York, 1966.

Heusinkveld, K. F., Cues to Communication with the Terminal Cancer Patient, *Nursing Forum*, 11, 1972, 105-112.

Johnson, B. S., The Meaning of Touch in Nursing, *Nursing Outlook*, 13, February 1965, 59-60.

Klagsburn, S. G., Communication in the Treatment of Cancer, *American Journal of Nursing*, 71(5), May 1971, 944-948.

Knapp, M. L., *Nonverbal Communications in Human Interaction*, 2nd ed., Holt, Rinehart & Winston, New York, 1978.

Krieger, D., Therapeutic Touch: The Imprimatur of Nursing, *American Journal of Nursing*, 75(5), May 1975, 784-787.

Kron, T., *Communication in Nursing,* Saunders, Philadelphia, 1972.

Kurtz, R., and Prestera, H., *The Body Reveals: An Illustrated Guide to the Psychology of the Body,* Harper & Row, New York, 1976.

LaFrance, M., and Mayo, C., *Moving Bodies—Nonverbal Communication in Social Relationships,* Brooks/Cole, Monterey, California, 1978.

Lewis, G. G., *Nurse-Patient Communication,* 2nd ed., Brown, Dubuque, Iowa, 1973.

McCorkle, R., Effects of Touch on Seriously Ill Patients, *Nursing Research,* 23(2), March–April 1974, 125–132.

Mehrabian, A., *Silent Messages,* Wadsworth, Belmont, California, 1971.

Mercer, L. S., Touch: Comforter or Threat? *Perspectives in Psychiatric Care,* 4, May–June 1966, 20–25.

Millar, D., and Millar, F., *Messages, Myths—Understanding Interpersonal Communication,* Knopf, New York, 1976.

Montagu, A., *Touching: The Human Significance of the Skin,* Columbia University Press, New York, 1971.

Mortensen, C. D., *Communication: The Study of Human Interaction,* McGraw-Hill, New York, 1972.

Mortensen, C. D., *Basic Readings in Communication Theory,* Harper & Row, New York, 1973.

O'Brien, M. J., *Communication and Relationships in Nursing,* Mosby, St. Louis, 1978.

Orlando, I., *The Dynamic Nurse-Patient Relationship,* Putnam's, New York, 1951.

Peplau, H., *Interpersonal Relations in Nursing,* Putnam's, New York, 1952.

Pluckhan, M. L., *Human Communication: The Matrix of Nursing,* McGraw-Hill, New York, 1978.

Rickelman, B. L., Bio-Psycho-Social Linguistics: A Conceptual Approach to Nurse-Patient Interaction, *Nursing Research,* 20(5), September–October 1971, 398–403.

Rubin, R., Body Image and Self Esteem, *Nursing Outlook,* 16(6), June 1968, 20–23.

Ruesch, J., and Kees, W., *Nonverbal Communication,* University of California Press, Los Angeles, 1972.

Schramm, W., *The Science of Human Communication,* Basic Books, New York, 1963.

Shannon, C., and Weaver, W., *The Mathematical Theory of Communication,* University of Illinois Press, Urbana, 1949.

Snyder, J. C., and Wilson, M. F., Elements of a Psychological Assessment, *American Journal of Nursing,* 77(2), February, 1977, 234–239.

Stetler, C. B., Relationship of Perceived Empathy to Nurses' Communication, *Nursing Research,* 26(6), November–December, 1977, 432–437.

Stewart, J., *Bridges Not Walls,* Addison-Wesley, Reading, Massachusetts, 1972.

Sweeney, M., Evaluating Nonverbal Skills of Nursing Students, *Journal of Nursing Education,* 16(3), March 1977, 5–11.

Thayer, L., *Communication and Communication Systems,* Irwin, Homewood, Illinois, 1968.

Topf, M., A Behaviroal Checklist for Estimating the Development of Communication Skills, *The Journal of Nursing Education,* 8, November 1969, 29–34.

Ujhely, G., Touch: Reflections and Perceptions, *Nursing Forum*, 18, 1979, 18-32.
Watzlawick, P., Beavin, J. H., and Jackson, D. D., *Pragmatics of Human Communication*, Norton, New York, 1967.
Weiss, S., The Language of Touch, *Nursing Research*, 28(2), March-April 1979, 76-79.
Wiener, N., *The Human Use of Human Beings*, Avon, New York, 1967.

## TRANSACTIONS

Anderson, N. L. An Interactive Systems Approach to Problem Solving, *The Nurse Practitioner*, 3(5), September-October 1978, 24-26.
Boulding, K., General Systems Theory—The Skeleton of Science, in *General Systems Yearbook*, edited by L. von Bertalanffy and A. Rapaport, vol. 1, Braun-Brumfield, Inc. Ann Arbor, Michigan, 1956, pp. 1-80.
Dewey, J., and Bentley, A., *Knowing and the Known*, Beacon Press, Boston, 1949.
Diers, D., and Schmidt, R., Interaction Analysis in Nursing Research, in *Nursing Research II*, edited by P. Verhonick, Little, Brown, Boston, 1977, pp. 77-132.
Grinker, R. (ed.), *Toward A Unified Theory of Human Behavior*, Basic Books, New York, 1967.
Howland, D., Models in Nursing Research, in *Nursing Research II*, edited by P. Verhonick, Little, Brown, Boston, 1977, 133-148.
Ittleson, W., and Cantril, H., *Perception: A Transactional Approach*, Doubleday, Garden City, New York, 1954.
Jones, E., and Thibaut, J. W., Interaction Goals as Bases of Inference in Interpersonal Perception, in *Person Perception and Interpersonal Behavior*, edited by R. Tagiuri and L. Petrullo, Stanford University Press, Palo Alto, California, 1958, 151-178.
Kelley, H., and Thibaut, J., *Interpersonal Relations: A Theory of Interdependence*, John Wiley & Sons, 1978.
King, I. M., *Toward a Theory for Nursing*, John Wiley & Sons, New York, 1971.
Kuhn, A., *Unified Social Science*, Dorsey Press, Homewood, Illinois, 1975.
Laing, R. D., Phillipson, H., and Lee, A. R., *Interpersonal Perception: A Theory and a Method of Research*, Harper & Row, New York, 1966.
Maxwell, C., Matter and Motion, in Dewey, J. and Bentley, A., *Knowing and the Known*, Beacon Press, Boston, 1949, p. 106, 107, 312.
Mead, G., *On Social Psychology: Selected Papers*, University of Chicago Press, Chicago, 1964.
Paterson, J., and Zderad, L. T., *Humanistic Nursing*, John Wiley & Sons, New York, 1976.
Rogers, C. R., *On Becoming a Person*, Houghton Mifflin, Boston, 1961.
Spiegel, J., *Transactions: The Interplay between Individual, Family, and Society*, Science House, New York, 1971.

Thibaut, J., and Jones, E., Interaction Goals as Bases of Inference in Interpersonal Perception, in *Person Perception and Interpersonal Behavior,* edited by R. Tagiuri and L. Petrullo, Stanford University Press, Palo Alto, California, 1958, 151-178.

Von Bertalanffy, L., *General System Theory: Foundations, Development and Application,* Braziller, New York, 1968.

Werley, H. H., Zuzich, A., Zajkowski, M., and Zagornik, A. D., *Health Research: The Systems Approach,* Springer, New York, 1976.

# ROLE

Arndt, C., and Laeger, E., Role Strain in a Diversified Role Set: The Director of Nursing Service, Part I, *Nursing Research,* 19(3), May-June, 1970, 253.

Backman, C., and Secord, P., The Self and Role Selection, in *The Self in Social Interaction,* edited by C. Gordon and K. J. Gergen, John Wiley & Sons, New York, 1968.

Benne, R. D., and Bennis, W. G., The Role of the Professional Nurse, *American Journal of Nursing,* 59(2), February 1959, 380-383.

Benner, R., and Kramer, M., Role Conceptions and Integrative Role Behavior of Nurses in Special Care and Regular Hospital Units, *Nursing Research,* 21(1), January-February 1972, 20-29.

Bevis, M. E., Role Conception and the Continuing Learning Activities of Neophyte Collegiate Nurses, *Nursing Research,* 22(3), May-June 1973, 207-216.

Brophy, E. B., Relationships among Self-Role Congruences and Nursing Experience, *Nursing Research,* 20(4), September-October 1971, 447-450.

Chaska, N. L., Status Consistency and Nurses' Expectations and Perceptions of Role Performance, *Nursing Research,* 27(6), November-December 1978, 356-364.

Corwin, R. G., The Professional Employee: A Study of Conflict in Nursing Roles, *American Journal of Sociology,* 66, 1961, 604.

Corwin, R. G., and Taves, M. J., Some Concomitants of Bureaucratic and Professional Conceptions of the Nurse Role, *Nursing Research,* 11(4), Fall 1962, 223-227.

Davis, A. J., Self-Concept, Occupational Role Expectations and Occupational Choice in Nursing and Social Work, *Nursing Research,* 19(1), January-February 1969, 55-50.

Dyer, E. D., Cope, M. J., Monson, M. A., and Von Drimmelen, J. B., Can Job Performance Be Predicted from Biographical, Personality, and Administrative Climate Inventories? *Nursing Research,* 21(4), July-August 1972, 294-304.

Folk-Lighty, M. A., and Brennan, A. M., Role Perception of the Staff Nurse in the Intensive Care Unit, *Heart & Lung,* 8(3), 1979, 535-539.

Gruendemann, B., Analysis of the Role of the Professional Staff Nurse in the Operating Room, *Nursing Research,* 19(4), July-August 1970, 349-350.

Haas, J. E., *Role Conception and Group Consensus: A Study of Disharmony in Hospital Work Groups,* Bureau of Business Research, College of Commerce and Administration, The Ohio State University, Columbus, Ohio, 1964.

Hadley, B. J., The Dynamic Interactionist Concept of Role, *The Journal of Nursing Education,* 6(2), April 1967, 5-25.

Hansen, A. C., and Upshaw, H. S., Evaluation within the Context of Role Analysis, *Nursing Research*, 11(3), Summer 1962, 144-150.

Hardy, M. E., and Conway, M. W., *Role Theory; Perspectives for Health Professionals*, Appleton-Century-Crofts, New York, 1978.

Hinshaw, A. S., and Field, M. A., An Investigation of Variables that Underlie Collegial Evaluation, *Nursing Research*, 23(4), July-August 1974, 292.

Hinshaw, A. S., and Oakes, D., Theoretical Model Testing: Patients', Nurses' and Physicians' Expectations for Quality Nursing Care, in *Communicating Nursing Research*, edited by M. Batey, WICHE, Boulder, Colorado, 1977, 163-191.

Kassebaum, G. G., and Baumann, B. O., Dimensions of the Sick Role in Chronic Illness, *Journal of Health and Human Behavior*, 6, 1974, 16-27.

Kellberg, E. B., Coronary Care Nurse Profile, *Nursing Research*, 21(1), January-February, 1972, 30-32.

Kramer, M., Role Models, Role Conceptions, and Role Deprivation, *Nursing Research*, 17(2), March-April 1968, 115-120.

Kramer, M., Role Conceptions of Baccalaureate Nurses and Success in Hospital Nursing, *Nursing Research*, 19(5), September-October 1970, 428-439.

Linton, R., *The Study of Man*, Appleton-Century-Crofts, New York, 1936.

Malone, M., Berkowitz, N., and Klein, M., Interpersonal Conflict in the Outpatient Department, *American Journal of Nursing*, 62(3), March 1962, 108.

Meleis, A. E., Role Insufficiency and Role Supplementation: A Conceptual Framework, *Nursing Research* 24(4), July-August 1975, 264-271.

Merton, R., *In Theoretical Sociology*, The Free Press, New York, 1967.

Minehan, P., Nurse Role Conception, *Nursing Research*, 26(5), September-October 1977, 374-379.

Parsons, T., *The Social System*, Free Press, Glencoe, Illinois, 1951.

Reich, S., and Geller, A., Self Image of Nurses, *Psychological Reports*, 39, 1979, 401-402.

Rubin, R., Attainment of the Maternal Role; Part II: Models and Referrents, *Nursing Research*, 16(5), Fall 1967, 343-346.

Schmitt, M., Role Conflict in Nursing—Is It Based on a Dubious Dichotomy? *American Journal of Nursing,* 68, November 1968, 2348-2350.

Skipper, J. K., Jr., and Leonard, R. C., *Social Interaction and Patient Care*, Lippincott, Philadelphia, 1965.

Smith, K., Discrepancies in the Role-Specific Values of Head Nurses and Nursing Educators, *Nursing Research*, 14(3), Summer 1965, 196-202.

Snyder, D. J., Role Conflict Is Here to Stay, *American Journal of Nursing*, 59(4), April 1969, 809-810.

# STRESS

Aiken, L. H., Systematic Relaxation to Reduce Preoperative Stress, *Canadian Nurse*, June 1972, 38-42.

Aiken, L. H., and Henrichs, T. F., Systematic Relaxation as a Nursing Intervention Technique with Open Heart Surgery Patients, *Nursing Research*, 20(3), May–June 1971, 212–217.

Anderson, M. S., and Pieticha, J. M., Emergency Unit Patients' Perceptions of Stressful Life Events, *Nursing Research*, 23(5), September–October 1974, 378–383.

Baughn, S. L., The Role of the Nurse in Dealing with Stress in the Industrial Setting, *Occupational Health Nursing*, 24, April 1976, 15–16.

Bell, J. M., Stressful Life Events and Coping Methods in Mental Illness and Wellness Behaviors, *Nursing Research*, 26(2), March–April 1977, 136–141.

Bellack, J. P., Helping a Child Cope with the Stress of Inquiry, *American Journal of Nursing*, 74(8), August 1974, 1491–1494.

Benson, H., Your Innate Asset for Combating Stress, *Psychology Today*, 8, February 1975, 33–34.

Breeden, S., and Kondo, C., Using Biofeedback to Reduce Tensions, *American Journal of Nursing*, 75(11), November 1975, 2010–2012.

Brink, P., Natural Triad in Health Care, *American Journal of Nursing*, 72(5), May 1972, 897–899.

Brockway, B., Plummer, O., and Lowe, B. M., Effect of Nursing Reassurance on Patient Vocal Stress Levels, *Nursing Research*, 25(6), November–December 1976, 440–445.

Brown, B., *New Mind, New Body*, Harper & Row, New York, 1974.

Brown, B., *Stress and the Art of Biofeedback*, Harper & Row, New York, 1977.

Cannon, W. B., *The Wisdom of the Body*, Norton, New York, 1963.

Cassem, N. Sources of Tension for the CCU Nurse, *American Journal of Nursing*, 72(8), August 1972, 1426–1430.

Castles, M. M., and Keith, P., Correlates of Environmental Fear in the Role of the Public Health Nurse, *Nursing Research*, 20(3), May–June 1971, 245–249.

Coombe, E. I., Tuning in on Stress Signals, *Journal of Nursing Education*, 15, July 1976, 16–21.

DeWalt, E., and Haines, S.A.K., The Effects of Specified Stressors on Healthy Oral Mucosa, *Nursing Research*, 18(1), January–February 1969, 22–27.

Dodge, D. L., and Martin, W. T., *Social Stress and Chronic Illness*, University of Notre Dame Press, South Bend, Indiana, 1970.

Dohrenwend, B. S., and Dohrenwend, B. P. (eds.), *Stressful Life Events: Their Nature and Effects*, John Wiley & Sons, New York, 1974.

Dumas, R., Utilization of Stress as a Therapeutic Nursing Measure, *ANA Clinical Sessions*, San Francisco, 1966, Appleton-Century-Crofts, New York, 1967.

Foster, S. B., An Adrenal Measure for Evaluating Nursing Effectiveness, *Nursing Research*, 23(2), March–April 1974, 118–124.

Friedman, E., Stress and the ICU Nurse, *Heart & Lung*, November–December 1972, 753–754.

Garret, A., Stressful Experiences Identified by Student Nurses, *Journal of Nursing Education*, 15, November 1976, 9–21.

Gentry, D., Anxiety and Urinary NA, K as Stress Indicators on Admission to CCU, *Heart & Lung*, November–December 1973, 875–877.

Gentry, D. W., Foster, S. B., and Froehling, S., Psychological Responses to Situational Stress in Intensive and Nonintensive Nursing, *Heart & Lung*, November–December 1972, 793–796.

Glass, D., Stress, Competition and Heart Attacks, *Psychology Toad*, 10, December 1976, 54–57.

Glass, D. S., and Singer, J. E., *Urban Stress*, Academic Press, New York, 1972.

Holmes, T. H., and Rahe, R. H., The Social Readjustment Rating Scale, *Journal of Psychosomatic Research*, 11, August 1967, 213–217.

Hunt, C., The Cause and Effect of Stress on Young People at Work, *Occupational Health Nursing*, 24, January 1976, 17–18.

Janis, I., *Psychological Stress*, John Wiley & Sons, New York, 1958.

Johnson, J. E., Effects of Structuring Patient Expectation on Their Reactions to Threatening Events, *Nursing Research*, 21(6), November–December 1972, 499–503.

Kicey, C. A., Catecholamines and Depression: A Physiological Theory of Depression, *American Journal of Nursing*, 74(11), November 1974, 2018–2020.

Kinsler, D., Relaxation: Key to Stress Reduction, *Occupational Health Nursing*, 25, July 1977, 7–8.

Leventhal, H., and Sharp, E., Facial Expressions as Indicators of Stress, in *Affect, Cognition and Personality*, edited by S. Tomkins and C. Izard, Springer, New York, 1965, p. 300.

Levine, S., and Scotch, N. A. (eds.), *Social Stress*, Aldine, Chicago, 1970.

McHenry, P., Contemporary Approach to Coronary Disease: Stress Testing in Coronary Heart Disease, *Heart and Lung*, January–February 1974, 83–92.

Marcinek, M. B., Stress in the Surgical Patient, *American Journal of Nursing*, 77(11), November 1977, 1809–1811.

Mechanic, D., *Students under Stress*, Free Press, Glencoe, Illinois, 1962.

Mechanic, D., Stress, Illness and Illness Behavior, *Journal of Human Stress*, 2(2), June 1976, 2–6.

Monat, A., and Lazarus, R. S. (eds.), *Stress and Coping*, Columbia University Press, New York, 1977.

Parisen, M. P., Rich, R., and Jackson, C. W., Suitability of the Subjective Stress Scale for Hospitalized Patients, *Nursing Research*, 18(6), November–December 1969, 529–533.

Pride, F. L., An Adrenal Stress Index as a Criterion Measure for Nursing, *Nursing Research*, 17(4), July–August 1968, 292–303.

Rabkin, J., and Struening, E., Life Events, Stress and Illness, *Science*, 194, December 1976, 1013–1020.

Schmitt, F., and Wooldridge, P. J., Psychological Preparation of Surgical Patients, *Nursing Research*, 22(2), March–April 1973, 108–116.

Schrodinger, E., *Space Time Structure*, University Press, Cambridge, England, 1950.

Scott, J., Stress and Coping: A Case for Intervention, *Journal of Psychiatric Nursing*, 15, February 1977, 14–17.

Sczekalla, R. M., Stress Reactions of CCU Patients and Resuscitative Procedures on Other Patients, *Nursing Research*, 22(1), January–February 1973, 65–70.

Sedgwick, R., Psychological Responses to Stress, *Journal of Psychiatric Nursing and Mental Health Services*, 13, September–October 1975, 20–23.

Selye, H., The Stress Syndrome, *American Journal of Nursing*, March 1965, 97–99.

Selye, H., A Code for Coping with Stress, *AORN Journal*, 25(1), January 1977, 35–42.

Seyle, H., *The Stress of Life*, McGraw-Hill, New York, 1956.

Seyle, H., *Stress without Distress*, Lippincott, Philadelphia, 1974.

Seyle, H., *Stress in Health and Disease*, Butterworths, Boston, 1975.

Slay, C., Myocardial Infarction and Stress, *The Nursing Clinics of North America*, 11(2), June 1976, 329–338.

Tooraen, L. A. Sr., Physiological Effects of Shift Rotation on ICU Nurses, *Nursing Research*, 21(5), September–October 1972, 398–405.

Visintainer, M. A., and Wolfer, J. A., Psychological Preparation for Surgical Pediatric Patients: The Effect on Children's and Parent's Stress Responses and Adjustment, *Pediatrics*, 56, August 1975, 187–202.

Volicer, B. J., Perceived Stress Levels of Events Associated with the Experience of Hospitalization, *Nursing Research*, 22(6), November–December 1973, 491–497.

Volicer, B. J., Patients Perceptions of Stressful Events Associated with Hospitalization, *Nursing Research*, 23(3), May–June 1974, 235–238.

Volicer, B. J., and Bohannon, M. W., A Hospital Stress Rating Scale, *Nursing Research*, 24(5), September–October 1975, 352–359.

Wolf, H. G., and Goodell, H., *Stress and Disease*, 2nd ed., Charles C Thomas, Springfield, Illinois, 1968.

# 4

# Social Systems

The nature of one's life in social groups tends to define the types of relationships that will be developed. Many social groups exist in different types of social systems. The pressures to conform to group goals and standards are strong. Reference groups tend to influence individuals' perceptions, judgments, and behavior. Social systems, such as the family, religious systems, educational systems, work systems, and peer groups, influence people as they grow, develop, and move from childhood to adulthood.

In daily associations with people from various cultural and socioeconomic groups, nurses have many opportunities to observe behavioral changes and their effect on themselves and others. Behavior results from learning experiences in the social systems in which individuals grow and develop their abilities to cope with change. The moving forces in nursing are imbedded in the dynamics of society in which the process of change alters the environment. Social forces are in constant motion within social systems, and the interplay of these forces influences social behavior, interactions, perceptions, and health.

There are social systems in which adults function as professionals, such as the hospital, public health agencies, industry, school, local, state, and national governments. The settings in which nurses deliver a service vary in size, structure, environment, values, resources, and goals. Nurses encounter a wide range of human experiences in the life cycle of human beings. Because of these factors, a construct of social systems is essential for a conceptual framework for nursing. The major concepts are organization, authority, power, status, and decision making. Common characteristics of each concept are discussed and terms defined. Implications for use of this knowledge in nursing are discussed.

## CHARACTERISTICS OF SOCIAL SYSTEMS

At birth, a person makes his debut into the first group, the family. The family is a social system because it exhibits such characteristics as structure, status, role, and social interaction. Within the family, beliefs, customs, and values are transmitted to the children. In most instances the family provides the initial process of socialization for the individual.

The biological inheritance of each person and the social systems into which a person is born, grows, and develops determine experiences and learning that influence behavior. Changes in human behavior are exhibited when individuals have acquired new knowledge or formed new insights based on previous knowledge or when there is some interference in the life cycle. Systems provide the framework for social interaction, define social relationships, and establish rules of behavior and modes of action. Beliefs, attitudes, values, and customs are learned within social systems, such as family, school, and church. Nurses, as individuals, are like all other human beings in this respect. They function within and are part of many different social systems.

Eisenstadt analyzed the difference between age groups by relating them to the structural characteristics of the social systems and their integrative mechanisms in order to demonstrate continuity in the systems. Some of these differences are the life span that the age groups cover, differences between task performance, and types of conformity or deviancy. "Age and differences of age are among the most basic and crucial aspects of human life and determinants of human destiny.... It becomes a basis for defining human beings, for the formation of mutual relationships and activities, and for the differential allocation of social roles" (Eisenstadt, 1964, p. 21). The problems of age are universal, whereas the process of aging is biologically and often culturally defined. The adult role is very distinctly defined in most societies. It is a time when individuals become full members of the social system of a community.

Analysis of the dynamics of social systems by Parsons showed the structural bases as the act, the status-role, and the individual actor who participates in a "patterned interactive relationship" (Parsons, 1951). The role and status of nurses in health care systems, such as staff nurse, supervisor, director of nursing, indicate some of the functional characteristics. In addition, as individuals, both the health clients and nurses have had different life experiences in various types of social systems. These factors influence behavior, beliefs, and the way in which people congnitively structure the world around them. As individuals nurses learn customs, attitudes, beliefs, and modes of behavior within institutions in the same way as the people for whom they provide professional services. However, the difference between nurses and clients is in the specialized knowledge skills, professional behaviors, and values that distinguish nurses and nursing.

Social class, role, status, and ethnic values appear to be critical variables that enter into perception and interaction. One of the first studies of the role of nurses indicated divergence in roles and expectations of individuals (Benne and Bennis, 1959).

Certain structural and functional characteristics are found in all social systems—values, behavior patterns, prescribed roles, status, authority, and age gradation. Linton compared the nature of a social system to a geometric figure—"a bit of nothing intricately drawn together." A social system is a configuration of relationships within a culture. Culture is a pattern of living, a way of behaving, thinking, believing, valuing, and feeling that is cumulative from one generation to another and that changes in the process of cross-cultural contact. Roles, status, and authority are part of the pattern of living. The settings in which nurses perform their functions exhibit these structural and functional characteristics. Knowledge of the influence of social systems on the behavior of individuals and groups is relevant for nurses.

## DEFINITION OF SOCIAL SYSTEM

A social system is defined as an organized boundary system of social roles, behaviors, and practices developed to maintain values and the mechanisms to regulate the practices and rules. Certain structural elements are defined in the type of formal and informal organization. Within the organization, certain functional elements are defined as prescribed roles, position, lines of authority and communication.

Concepts of organization, power, authority, status, and decision making are characteristics of social systems that have relevance for nursing.

## Concept of Organization

Individuals spend most of their waking life in organizations. The organizational environments provide some of the social forces that mold and develop personal qualities and habits. The parameters in any organization are: (1) human values, behavior patterns, needs, goals and expectations; (2) a natural environment in which material and human resources are essential for achieving goals; (3) employers and employees or parents and children, who form the groups that collectively interact to achieve goals; (4) technology that facilitates goal attainment.

If individuals spend a good portion of their adult life in work situations called organizations, it is helpful to understand the organizational environment. One approach to the analysis of the total organization is the use of the following criteria:

1. What is the philosophy of the organization? For example, what beliefs are held about people, about products, about power and authority?
2. What are the goals of the organization? Do these goals reflect a concern not only for organizational goals but also for individual and group goals?
3. What are the functions of the organization?
4. What are the resources of the organization?
5. What are some of the constraints in the organization?
6. Who makes the decisions at all levels of the organization?

### CHARACTERISTICS OF ORGANIZATION

Organizations are social units characterized by structure, functions, and resources to achieve goals.

The structure of an organization provides for an ordering of positions and activities that include size, complexity, formal and informal arrangements. Since the industrial revolution, formal organizations have developed because of increased dependency of people upon each other for survival. As business and industry expanded, organizations became a way of economy and efficiency in productivity and in profit. Early studies of organization tried to find ways to minimize costs and maximize profits. Formal organizations were developed that provided a division of labor, span of control, organized structure, authority, and decision making within the organization. Formal organizations provide the framework, positions, procedures, and tasks for assigning specific activities to each position with prescribed rules and regulations.

In recent years people interested in human relations in organizations have provided for individual workers and organizations to achieve goals. The informal structure has accomplished some gains for individuals in the formal system. The term *informal* refers to natural grouping of people in a work situation to meet individual and group needs not met by the formal organization. Informal organizations are characterized by who talks with whom, by an informal communication system sometimes called the grapevine, by social control and emergence of an informal leader, by coping with change, by meeting basic needs, by recognition in the work situation. The informal structure is made up of groups with common interests who develop their own norms and relations within the formal organization. Some of the differences between formal and informal organizations are:

| *Formal* | *Informal* |
|---|---|
| Division of labor | Personal needs and interests are the basis for groups forming |
| Chain of command | |
| Positions with control, power, authority | Group norms for behavior emerge |
| Primary goal to achieve outcomes of organization | Primarily formed to meet personal needs |
| Formal leader, such as supervisor | Informal leader emerges from the group |
| Subordinates in prescribed roles | Members by choice |

Structure relates to the formal and informal arrangements of individuals and groups to achieve individual and organizational goals. This idea of an organization has been called a traditional type of organization or the classical or neoclassical type. The most recent studies and writings about organizations refer to a systems approach that stems from operational research and systems analysis. McDonough and Garrett (1965, p. 17) noted a few differences between the old and new look in organizations:

| *Classical or Neoclassical* | *Systems* |
|---|---|
| 1. Emphasizes design of organizational structure and then | 1. Emphasizes the design of communication and interac- |

| *Classical or Neoclassical* | *Systems* |
|---|---|
| thinks about the communication and interactions needed to achieve goals. | tions and then thinks about organizational strucuture to achieve goals. |
| 2. Emphasizes the chain of command, authority, and responsibility. | 2. Emphasizes channels of communication, information flow, and decisions. |
| 3. Provides compartments of authority and responsibility. | 3. Provides networks between question and answer points. |

In a systems approach to organization theory the concepts are identified as: (1) elements that are individuals, structure, roles, norms, and physical environment; (2) interrelationships of units to accomplish goals of organization and of individual members; (3) information and communication processes; (4) growth and viability through feedback; and (5) decision making, implementation, and evaluation.

Structure identifies functions, which is the second characteristic of organization. Functions are identified with roles, position, and activities to be performed. Some functions are decision making, assignment of tasks to specific people, recruitment and maintenance of human resources, training and socialization, design and implementation of rewards and fringe benefits. In organizations that deliver social services as a primary goal, overall functions and material resources are identified, but when professionals are involved in the delivery of services, expertise is required to achieve specific goals of the organization. In health care organizations functions and human resources are related to goals, which is the third characteristic.

Goals are identified as the outcomes to be achieved. In some organizations, the goals are the production, marketing, and selling of a product. In some organizations, the primary goal is providing human services such as health care. For these latter organizations that provide health care services, the goal is helping individuals maintain their health, regain it if they have had some disturbance in their health, prevent recurrence of illness and disease, if possible, and learn to cope with chronic illness or disease. In health care organizations, it is important to recognize the need for professionals to achieve their goals, if optimal and effective service is to be expected. Individuals in organizations have demonstrated greater efficiency and satisfaction when they participate in decisions about goals and then agree to the means to achieve personal and organizational goals.

From these characteristics derived from studies and organization theories, a definition can be formulated.

**Definitions of organization.** Individuals and groups are the social units of an organization. An organization is a system whose continuous activities are conducted to achieve goals. In this system of activities, the roles of individuals depict the human elements of complex interrelated systems in organizations.

DiVincenti defined organization as "a configuration of people and resources put together in a manner apparently best suited to achieve particular objectives" (DiVincenti, 1972, p. 46). Organizations accomplish purposes through groups (Katz and Kahn, 1966).

An operational definition is suggested. *An organization is composed of human beings with prescribed roles and positions who use resources to accomplish personal and organizational goals.*

## IMPLICATIONS FOR NURSING

For the past 30 years, organizations in the United States have increased in complexity and in their influence on other social systems, such as the family. Psychologists, sociologists, and managers have described, explained, and even predicted effects of the organization on people's lives and on human values. Since nurses provide their services in a variety of health care organizations, and since the consumers they serve have been influenced by the organizations in which they have grown and developed, knowledge of a concept of organization is essential in educating nurses for the future.

Organizational structure, which is often shown in an organizational chart, specifies relationships, lines of authority, communication, responsibility, and positions related to specific functions. Most nurses are employed in formal organizations. In the role of nurse, there is potential conflict as one is responsible for functioning to achieve the goals of the organization and also the goals of professional nursing. It is important for nurses to understand formal organizations in order to function within them and to assume professional responsibility for their functions as well as to assume accountability to the institution. Above all, the nurse is accountable to the person who receives the nursing care.

Within hospital organizations there are many subunits that influence care of persons. Professionals and technicians are responsible for x-rays, physical therapy, and laboratory tests. The formal organization demands that nurses coordinate most of the functions of others that are related to patients in hospitals. It is important for nurses to understand the informal system, the grapevine. It is important to understand departmental territory and role relationships. When one understands the lines of communication and interacts with people directly and in written memos, clarity of information and accuracy in perceptions are maintained.

Satisfaction of the member of an organization is important. When it is not present, high turnover, low morale, and high sickness and accident rates may result. High turnover means loss of money, which means poor use of resources.

Nurses have a crucial role to play in health care organizations as active participants in making decisions that influence the quality of care. Serving on committees gives nurses opportunities to assert leadership and to bring institutional, individual, and professional goals into balance and harmony.

Understanding of formal and informal organizations can help nurses identify and deal with conflict between the organization and professional roles and functions. Effective decision making is a key to organizational survival and productivity. For example, high turnover of nurses in hospitals is costly and at times indicates low morale. This may also mean that nurses' goals and needs are not being met by the organization. Satisfaction is predicted if administrators in an organization encourage participation in decision making that affects the employees. When nurses can clearly articulate their roles and functions as professionals and demonstrate little conflict in hospitals, nursing care will improve in quality.

Nurses are the only health group that provide constancy and continuity in a variety of organizations, such as schools, industry, official and voluntary health agencies at the local, state, and national level, and hospitals of different sizes, controls, and resources, which employ more than 50 percent of practicing nurses. Other professionals move in and out of health care systems. The recent additions to the variety of systems are nursing homes, extended care facilities, ambulatory care, neighborhood health clinics, crises centers, and drug and alcohol centers.

Hospitals are systems of many interrelated and interdependent departments. Nurses are asked to coordinate patient care activities around various department goals and functions, which often creates conflict. Nurses are expected to supervise nonprofessional care givers, which may cause frustration if the supervisory and coordinating aspects of the role detract from the clinical practice role. Nurses are coordinators by default because they are the only group in the hospital that is continuously present in patient care units 24 hours a day and 7 days a week. This expectation by hospital administrators and directors of nursing may cause conflict and dissatisfaction by taking the nurse away from performing the functions of professional nursing. If nurses are expected to continue in the role of coordinator in health care systems such as hospitals, then they should have some formal education to prepare them for this role.

Knowledge of organizations can assist nurses in the way they influence change in health care systems. They do this by serving on committees in the organization, such as quality assurance and PSRO committees, infection control, policies, procedures, and research committees.

An organization is made up of individuals and groups with prescribed roles, norms, values, all structured to achieve goals. If nurses are to perform their functions as professionals, they must influence the organization to achieve standards whereby quality care can be measured.

Nurses must be aware of crisis administration in which they are asked to work because it is difficult to maintain professional standards and provide quality care when the organization is in constant upheaval and changes are made with no participation by those whom the changes will affect. Decision making at all levels of the organization influences the delivery of nursing care. Nurses must be able to participate in decisions related to their role and functions.

Suggestions for successful functioning in a health care organization are:

1. Assess the organization, using objective criteria, to determine if your professional and personal goals can mesh with the organizational goals.
2. Agree with the written philosophy and its implementation.
3. Agree with the goals of the organizations.
4. Know who makes decisions that affect care.
5. Identify the lines of formal and informal communication and the power.
6. Assess the kind of management that prevails, such as participative type or autocratic type.

Organization as a system exhibits patterns of individual and group behavior, patterns of communication, and patterns of interaction related to role. Interactive patterns of behavior are related to subconcepts of organization, such as authority, power, and status.

## Concept of Authority

Authority is power to make decisions that guide the actions of self and others. If A perceives B as one who may legitimately make decisions, then B has authority over A. Most people define authority as that power one has in holding a certain position, such as that of judge, supervisor, director of nursing, hospital administrator. Individuals in these positions may or may not exert leadership.

All human beings experience some dependence on authority at different points in their life. In the course of growth and development, human beings move from dependency in childhood to independence and interdependence in adulthood. In some individuals an early pattern of dependency was never resolved, and as adults they feel comfortable and secure in relations that continue the pattern. When these individuals become administrators, authority problems may exist in the organization, such as inability to make decisions.

Authority can be divided into two types: formal and functional. Proponents of formal authority have been Weber, Taylor, Urich, and Gulich. This conventional approach to authority is characterized by formal, rational, and impersonal behaviors. Weber viewed authority as legal-rational, traditional, and charismatic. Legal-rational authority offered norms and rules in which persons by their position had certain rights. Traditional authority espoused established practices and the right of descendents to exercise authority, such as the right of kings. Charismatic authority was derived from knowledge, or from personal experience and achievements (Weber, 1947).

Taylor (1947) believed authority resided in the techniques of scientific management. Gulich (1937) believed that authority came from those with expert knowledge. Authority is "legitimate power" given to a person by virtue of role and position in a social system (Katz and Kahn, 1966).

Authority is observed all around us in various situations: teacher-student, mother-child, employer-employee.

Simon (1962) stated that authority most be looked at from the point of view of sanctions and rewards, legitimization, technical skills, and social approval as a basis for acceptance of authority. Barnard (1954) discussed acceptance of authority based on the perceptions of persons. He indicated that: (1) individuals are willing to accept another's control without conscious questioning; (2) individuals make decisions as to whether they will or will not be influenced by another; or (3) individuals refuse to recognize authority of another and reject it.

Authority is seen by some as residing in the role and position in a formal organization and by others as residing in the person by virtue of knowledge and expertise, such as the authority of a professional.

## CHARACTERISTICS OF AUTHORITY

In every society or culture, authority can be observed as it provides order, guidance, and responsibility for actions. All individuals are subject to authority in the maintenance of order and safety in a society. In this sense, authority is universal.

Authority is essential in formal organizations. It guides and directs behavior in an organization. It is reciprocal because it takes two individuals for authority to exist, one who influences another and the other who accepts that influence. It requires that individuals cooperate in an organization or a society to achieve goals and to maintain order and peace. In situations where authority is exerted, there is at least one person who is superior, with authority, and one who is subordinate. This type of authority is expected to result in cooperation and communication in an organization.

Before authority can be exercised in any situation, a person must be perceived as having legitimate authority. This perception is situational. For example, a nurse's aide may perceive a head nurse as having authority by virtue of knowledge, skills, and position in a hospital. Outside of that organization and situation, the perception of the nurse as a person in another situation may be different. Authority is a function of concrete situations in which one person commands and one obeys and functions change as situations change. One may accept an authority figure in a crisis and reject the same person when the crisis abates.

Authority is essential to the achievement of goals. It is used to coordinate and regulate behaviors to achieve goals. It is one way to try to assure role expectations and performance in a position.

Power is a characteristic of authority. In formal organizations, authority gives power to regulate and to enforce rules or norms, thus controlling people's behavior to gain their cooperation in the achievement of goals. This control implies a superior–subordinate relationship among individuals in the organization and acceptance by the subordinate.

## DEFINITION OF AUTHORITY

From publications on the topic of authority, authority can be said: (1) to be legitimate and perceived by individuals; (2) to reside in the position held by a person who distributes the sanctions and the rewards; (3) to reside in the competence of a person with special knowledge and skills, such as professionals; and (4) to reside in the person who uses human relations skills to exercise leadership in a group.

Authority is a transactional process characterized by active, reciprocal relations in which members' values, background, and perception play a role in defining, validating, and accepting the authority of individuals within an organization. One person influences another, and he recognizes, accepts, and complies with the authority of that person.

## IMPLICATIONS FOR NURSING

In some form every society demonstrates some type of authority. For example, one accepts the norms and values of society or is subject to sanctions of that society. In most instances, the authority of parents, teachers, employers, or religious leaders is accepted by individuals and groups in a variety of organizations. Authority can be observed when one person or group accepts and follows the command and behavior of another person or group. Authority is seen as a relationship of individuals in an organization to achieve goals.

Authority is not a quality that some people have and others do not possess. It is an interrelationship between actor and acted upon. It is reciprocal because each is dependent upon the other; the superior who issues the command or makes the decision depends upon the subordinate to follow the command or implement the decision.

It is essential that nurses understand their position in an organization, the power and authority of the position, and the delegation of decision making in the organization. Appropriate use of the lines of authority and the channels of communication in formal organizations serve both the individual and the organization. The formal system provides for achievement of organizational goals and personal and professional goals.

Hospitals are forms of hierarchical organizations in which there are superiors and subordinates in terms of line and staff positions. However, authority in nursing in hospitals presents a two-sided picture. Nurses have legal authority (or legitimate authority) by virtue of their license to practice the profession of nursing. The hospital delegates authority to supervisors and other management personnel to make decisions that affect the functions of nurses. If nurses are placed in supervisory positions and have the authority to hire and fire, to promote and increase salaries, and to evaluate performance and effectiveness of care given by other nurses, conflict may arise. There may be no acceptance of the authority of the supervisor in terms of quality care, but there may be an acceptance because of the power to administer sanctions and rewards. This duality of authority as a professional with legitimate authority and in a subordinate role in which nurses are placed in the hierarchical structure of hospitals can do nothing but cause frustration and high turnover unless nurses exercise their legitimate authority in the area of professional nursing care.

In the various health care systems in which nurses work, they must understand the lines of authority in the organization as well as their legitimate authority by virtue of being a professional. Only when nurses understand authority will they be able to function effectively in an organization. For example, the department of nursing in hospitals should have equal status with all other departments and should have the authority to make decisions for nursing. Only nurses can speak with authority about nursing, its roles, functions, and responsibilities. Yet, one of the most subtle administrative techniques used in hospitals is to cut the budget of the department of nursing which indicates that the person who controls the budget exerts the power and authority in the organization. Nurses speak with authority about the legal and ethical responsibilities in nursing.

Independent functions of nurses are those for which they have authority by law and are accountable for performing. Collaborative functions are those in which nurses and physicians work together to achieve the goals of patient care.

The clinical specialist role in a hospital is an example of use of authority. When placed in a staff position, a clinical specialist functions as an expert practitioner and staff educator. Without some authority in the formal organization, the clinical specialist role may be difficult and frustrating as there is no authority in the position to influence the quality of nursing care. The clinical specialist's expertise as one type of authority is ineffective in a hospital without some position in which authority is perceived by staff nurses and is followed in the delivery of nursing care. If the clinical specialist is expected to demonstrate changes in nursing care, then authority must be perceived when necessary in the decisions made to provide effective nursing care.

Appropriate use of authority in an organization promotes worker satisfaction, efficiency, high morale, and achievement of goals.

## Concept of Power

A concept of power is closely related to authority. In any organization one will see the influence and/or effects of power. Power in social life is analogous to energy in the physical world. Both are discussed, but cannot be directly observed or measured. Their existence and strength are inferred from their effects. Power is seen in the role one enacts and in the positions one occupies. Although power exists within social relationships, the individuals who exercise it can control groups, organizations, and nations.

Power is an essential element in social systems. Several uses of power have been discussed, such as decision making, dominance over information, control of the budget, persuasion, deprivation, or compensation.

Influence is an instance of power in which outcomes are not predetermined. Peer groups exert power over individuals, which may be seen as a type of force. Control is an instance of power in which outcomes are usually predetermined. For example, if one controls the amount of money that can be spent for a particular piece of equipment, this control leaves little doubt about outcome. Use of strikes by unions and organizations is an instance of power. Power exists in relation to a situation or an organization.

### CHARACTERISTICS OF POWER

Power is universal in that all individuals and organizations experience power either as the one controlling events or the one being controlled. Power is felt in families, in schools, in relations with individuals and in political systems.

Power is situational. Power is not a personal attribute although individuals have some control over some events in their lives. In one situation a person may have legitimate power and exercise it; in another situation the same person is powerless. Power implies a dependency relationship as seen in the superior–subordinate role. Exertion of power by one person is dependent on the acceptance of that power by another person. Power is essential in an organization for the maintenance of balance and harmony. However, misuse of power may cause chaos and disorganization. Power is limited by the resources in a situation.

Power is dynamic. Events and people are continuously changing. Power is seen as losses and gains in life. Power is having some control over the process of change in an organization.

Power is *goal directed.* Appropriate use of power will help individuals achieve goals. If there are no goals, there is no power. Power is a means for organizations to implement decisions.

The nature of power can be seen in the following premises:

1. Power is potential energy.
2. Power is essential for order in society.
3. Power enhances group cohesiveness.
4. Power resides in positions in organizations.
5. Power is directly related to authority.
6. Power is a function of human interactions.
7. Power is the function of decision making.

Power is the capacity to use resources in organizations to achieve goals.

## DEFINITION OF POWER

Power is the process whereby one or more persons influence other persons in a situation. Power defines a situation in a way that people will accept what is being done while they may not agree with it.

Griffiths (1959) indicated that power is a function of decision making, and defined it as $P = f(D)$. The person who has the most control over the decision-making process in an organization has the most power. The ability of a person to achieve a goal has implied that motivation factors provide personal power.

Power is an ability to control events and behaviors in specific situations. Etzioni (1975) noted that power is an ability to reduce resistance and to make changes in a field over a period of time. Katz and Kahn (1966) defined power as the capacity to exert influence over people and situations. Zald (1970) noted that power is intentional control over individuals and groups, which influences goal attainment.

Power is the capacity or ability of a person or a group to achieve goals; power occurs in all aspects of life and each person has potential power determined by individual resources and the environmental forces encountered. Power is social force that organizes and maintains society. Power is the ability to use and to mobilize resources to achieve goals. Power may guide, direct, control, and change the behavior of individuals and groups. Power is the energy of the organization.

## IMPLICATIONS FOR NURSING

When one possesses power in an organization, one can control resources and access to information and to people. When individuals believe they can influence change in an organization or a system and implement a plan for change, they are exercising power. If those individuals in the organization perceive this plan as one that meets their needs, they will help implement the change. This is acceptance of power. Until recently, nurses have not been aware of their power as individuals or as a unified group within a professional organization that provides collective power for nurses.

In the past, nurses have been subjected to the use of power by individuals and organizations who made decisions about health care. Nurses have recently begun to exercise their power by virtue of their knowledge, skills, and expertise in meeting health care needs of people. Power is inherent in decisions made by nurses that influence the care of individuals in health care systems. The potential power of nurses has not been demonstrated in the United States. As the largest group numerically in the country, nurses have the potential power to influence the quality of health care but they have not unified their collective power to influence decision making about health care in local, state, and federal governments. Can you imagine what would happen if one million nurses would write letters to their elected officials about a major issue, such as national health insurance?

The nursing profession cannot use power unless it agrees on a set of unified goals as a basis for group action. As individuals, nurses may have little power to influence national decisions, but as a group of professionals the potential power is an untapped source of influence on health policies. As individuals nurses can demonstrate power when they interact with patients mutually to set goals and agree to the means to achieve them.

Recognition that power is related to support and respect of others will help nurses support and respect the clients served. Power is potential energy to be used for effective action in organizations.

The use of power in society is called politics. Politics means the process through which social power is distributed and exercised, with emphasis on collective decisions. Power protects relationships among people to maintain order and to achieve goals. Power is a means of getting the essential resources that help to produce efficiency in an organization. Power provides for goal achievement. Status influences the acceptance of power.

## Concept of Status

Status in an organization is one dimension of stratification. Sociologists have indicated that position determines a nurse's status in health care systems. Status is the position of an individual in a group as perceived by other individuals in the group. Status is the prestige attached to role. For example, the nurse role has more prestige than the aide's role and is viewed as having higher status.

Linton (1963) described status as ascribed or achieved. Achieved status is gained through individual choice and through one's abilities, performance, and skills. Ascribed status is determined by birth, such as sex, race, social class, and religion.

### CHARACTERISTICS OF STATUS

Status is situational. A father and mother in a family have status but as members of an art class have no status. A student may have status because of his rank in class or his achievement generally but no status as an athlete.

Status depends on position. One is perceived to have status when in positions valued by some individuals as high in status. One has status by virtue of socioeconomic class in society.

Status is reversible. One may hold a position of status and resign that position. The status goes with the position. When a person loses his place in an organization that was perceived by others to have prestige, he loses status in the organization.

### DEFINITION OF STATUS

Status is defined as the position of an individual in a group or a group in relation to other groups in an organization. Status has accompanying privileges, duties, and obligations. Status is that which is attached to role or position. Status is one dimension of social stratification. Status is related to who you are, what you do, who you know, and what you have achieved.

**IMPLICATIONS FOR NURSING**

Nurses should be able to recognize status in an organization and to identify those individuals who have a need for status. An example of a person who has a need for status is one who uses three or four degrees or titles behind his signature. Some indivdauls in health care systems are so status-conscious that they demand to be called by certain titles.

On the other hand, nurses must recognize the importance of status in situations which influence goal attainment. For example, the way you address your congressman may determine whether or not he will respond to you. These individuals make decisions that influence the status of nurses economically.

Nursing in hospitals has historically had a status stratification. For example, nurses have been given titles such as supervisor, head nurse, director of nursing, clinician 1, 2, 3, 4 and all imply status. Nurses must be aware of individuals in an organization who will listen only to people they perceive to have status, and use this awareness to achieve goals. Recognition of the status needs of patients in hospitals is essential to give effective nursing care. Status is associated with individuals who have the power and authority to make decisions.

# Concept of Decision Making

Every day decisions are being made that affect how individuals act and what is expected of them as human beings. Decisions are the judgments made that affect a course of action to be taken in specific situations. In organizations, decisions are made at every level of the structure. Decision making is a key concept in any organization. In reflecting on the process of decision making, choice and action enter into the judgment.

Decision making has become an increasingly more important concept for all people in all aspects of life. It has become extremely important in the health field and the lives of health clients and families, nurses and physicians.

Bross believed that a decision is "a process of selecting one action from a number of alternative courses of action" (Bross, 1953, p. 1). Young (1968) believed that criteria should be established to choose a course of action from among many alternatives and based on quantitative data analysis. Simon was the first to propose that decisions are not only based on facts but are influenced by value judgments as seen in the selection of goals to be achieved in an organization. Facts and values enter into decisions (Simon, 1957). As an organization becomes complex and expands, it increases the complexity of decisions to be made.

Simon (1957) described steps in decision making: (1) intellectual activity that establishes goals and priorities; (2) design activity that identifies alternative courses of action; (3) choice activity that is selecting an alternative and making a commitment; (4) implementation of choice; (5) evaluation of achievement of goals.

The use of operations research has influenced decision making by managers in organizations. Operations research involves the use of scientific method to study alternatives of a problem, and provides a quantitative basis for arriving at an optimum solution in terms of goals. Models are used to represent the interrelationship of variables. The simplest mathematical model that shows the relationship between two variables and a goal is: $E = f(x,y)$, where $E$ is the goal and $x$ is the course of action variable and $y$ is the background variable, which may not be controlled, and $f$ is the functional relationship between $x$ and $y$.

Shaefer (1974) related decision making and nursing process, and agreed with others that it is a choice subsequent to deliberation and judgment. Grier (1976) shared similar ideas about decision making in noting that decisions are influenced by many variables and should be guided by scientific principles and judgment in selection and implementation of actions to achieve specific goals.

There are at least three components in every decision: (1) the process, (2) the decision maker, and (3) the decision that is made. Decision making is defined as a process of choosing one alternative from many based on facts and values, implementation of the decision, and evaluation of achievement of goals. Decisions regulate activities in an organization and in one's life.

Decision making has been called the central process in administration, the core of planning, the heartbeat of the organization's activities, the key to good management, resolution of alternative choices, selection of a course of action, and an act of judging between alternatives based on analysis of consequences.

Decision theory identified components of the decision process as a set of alternatives or actions, outcomes associated with each alternative, probability of each outcome occurring, and the value of the outcome in relation to goals.

## CHARACTERISTICS OF DECISIONS

Decisions regulate each person's life and work. All human beings make decisions. Behavior is a result of decisions. Decisions are usually based on one's values, goals, knowledge, and past experience. Decisions are individual, personal, and subjective.

Decisions are situational. The contect in which a decision is made is related to goals and the specific situation. Decisions are influenced by timing, the amount of information available, and the persons involved. Perceptions of the decision maker influence choice of alternatives.

Decision making is a continuous process. In the course of analyzing facts gathered to make rational decisions, a continuous process is observed in interpretation of the facts, in relationship of facts to values and goals. It is a dynamic, ongoing process in life and in organizations. When a choice is made to implement a specific decision, many more decisions must be made. It is like problem solving; when one problem has been solved, it raises many more questions to be answered.

Decisions are goal-directed. Most decisions in organizations are made on the basis of the objective of the organization. A purposeful and conscious process is engaged in where those responsible for decisions identify and clarify the goal, select from several alternatives an approach that has few consequences, and assess probability that goals can be accomplished. Decisions may be altered on the basis of new information or new goals. The idea in decision making is to select a course of action that can be completed in the shortest amount of time and with the least amount of money and energy but with the best outcomes.

## DEFINITION OF DECISION MAKING

*Decision making in organizations is a dynamic and systematic process by which goal-directed choice of perceived alternatives is made and acted upon by individuals or groups to answer a question and attain a goal.*

The decision-making process involves a situation, a state of affairs, or a problem. Decision making is defining the problem, analyzing the facts gathered, and selecting the best alternative course of action in terms of goals by weighing risks against gains, economy of effort, time, and limitation of resources. The decision is translated into a plan for action. Those individuals who are expected to implement a decision should participate in making it and in formulating the plans.

Effectiveness of decisions are evaluated in terms of goal attainment or problems resolved with the least amount of dollars spent, the least amount of energy used, and the least amount of disturbance in the organization.

## IMPLICATIONS FOR NURSING

Provisions for direct and indirect nursing care require decisions about goals to be achieved in each nurse-client situation and in each family situation. When nurses engage in mutual goal setting with health clients they help them make decisions and choose between alternatives in their care.

The decision-making process requires information. In patient care situations in hospitals, this need for information means nurses give information to patients and patients share information with nurses. Both can withhold information, but this procedure would not be advantageous in making decisions about goals to be attained. Sharing information with patients does not imply that nurses have the right to reveal information of a medical nature that is the prerogative of the physician.

The computer age and new information systems will be helpful in storing and retrieving data of a decision-making nature in nursing practice. Currently, nurses use very few information forms that provide the kind of recordings about nursing care that can be stored and retrieved.

A theory for nursing in the next chapter is derived from the conceptual framework. A goal-oriented nursing record lends itself to computerization of accurate data gathered by nurses, and can be used mutually to set goals with patients, to identify nursing problems, and to move to transactions that indicate the goals that were achieved. This record can be separately used but should be used in conjunction with Weed's Problem Oriented Medical Record. The decisions of the nurses and of the physicians will be recorded on the same record so that comparisons can be made between medical care and nursing care. In order to use this kind of record, nurses must have knowledge, skills, and the ability to articulate clearly and concisely the nursing care they are giving by using a systematic data base from which nurses record a nursing problem list and a nursing goal list. This record system will show that quality assurance in nursing includes process and outcomes based on a theory of transactions.

Use of POMR and GONR would improve medical diagnosis and nursing diagnosis and would demonstrate effectiveness of patient care on the basis of goals attained.

Shaeffer noted that "the client becomes the connecting link between the decision making process and the nursing process" (Shaeffer, 1974, p. 1853). Nurses must be conscious of the patients' rights to make decisions and offer information that may be helpful in selecting alternative courses of action.

Hammond and Kelly's study of clinical inference noted that the multiple variables surrounding each nursing situation are complex and the number of decision making events and kinds of decisions nurses were expected to make were complex (Kelly, 1966). Hansen and Thomas's study to conceptualize decision making produced a model that included situational variables, contextual variables, and decision-maker variables (Hansen and Thomas, 1970). A few studies about decision making have shown the complexity and variability in each situation nurses encounter in hospitals and in the community.

Decision makers are usually perceived to have power and authority and tend to control decisions. Kelly noted that "in the performance of her professional duties the nurse routinely makes important decisions based on uncertain data—data that are complex, nondiscriminating and inconclusive" (Kelly 1964, p. 314).

Human life is a continuous decision-making process. In life and death situations in health care systems, knowledge and skills in decision making are essential for all health care professionals.

Decisions about patient care in hospitals are often made unilaterally by a nurse or a physician. Information is shared by nurses who interact with patients, and decisions are made about priorities of goals and the means to achieve them. Factors in the environment that influence these decisions may be classified as *situational variables*. Nurses' and patients' variables are related to their knowledge, background of experience, goals, values, and perceptions of the situation.

The source of information in a hospital is the patient. Another source of information is the knowledge the professional brings to the situation. When information is shared between patient and professional, informed decisions can be made about a course of action. When individuals participate in the decisions that will influence their lives, there is less resistance to implementing those decisions, and learning takes place.

Nurses should be aware of the patient's need for help in making decisions and need to share in those decisions. Nurse educators must prepare the future generation of nurses to make decisions in nursing situations. The influence of social systems on the decision-making process at all levels of organization can enhance or detract from effectiveness of care.

## Summary

Knowledge of the influence of social systems on the behavior of individuals and groups is relevant for nurses. Nurses have multiple opportunities to function in diverse settings, and to be effective in their professional roles they must have an understanding of the background of individuals in social systems and of the health care systems within which they function.

Nurses are expected to synthesize knowledge from natural and behavioral sciences, and to use knowledge in making decisions in immediate life-and-death situations. Nurses are expected to share knowledge with patients to help them learn ways to cope with illness and chronic health problems. One way to achieve health goals is through human interactions of consumers and health professionals.

Human beings are continuously interacting with other human beings and objects in their environment. Nurses and patients in hospitals are human beings who interact in specific situations for specific purposes. A theory of goal attainment that describes, explains, and may predict outcomes in nurse-patient interactions is proposed in the next chapter.

## Bibliography

### ORGANIZATION

Abrahamson, M. (ed.), *The Professional in the Organization,* Rand McNally, Chicago, 1967.

Argyris, G., *Interpersonal Competence and Organizational Effectiveness,* Irwin-Dorsey, Homewood, Illinois, 1962.

Arndt, C., and Huckabay, L., *Nursing Administration: Theory for Practice with a Systems Approach,* Mosby, St. Louis, 1980.

Barnard, C., *The Functions of the Executive,* Harvard University Press, Cambridge, Massachusetts, 1954.

Benne, R. D., and Bennis, W. G., The Role of the Professional Nurse, *American Journal of Nursing,* 59(2), February 1959, 380-383.

Bennis, W. G., Benne, K. D., and Chin, R., *The Planning of Change,* Holt, Rinehart & Winston, New York, 1969.

Blau, P., *On the Nature of Organizations,* John Wiley & Sons, New York, 1974.

Coffey, R., Athos, A., and Raynolds, P., *Behavior in Organizations: A Multidimensional View,* Prentice-Hall, Englewood Cliffs, New Jersey, 1975.

Cooley, C. H., *Social Organization,* Schocken Books, New York, 1972.

Cyert, R. M., and March, J. G., Organizational Goals, in *Groups and Organizations,* edited by B. Hinton and J. Reitz, Wadsworth, Belmont, California, 1969.

Divincenti, M., *Administering Nursing Service,* Little, Brown, Boston, 1977.

Durbin, R. L., and Springall, H. W., *Organization and Administration of Health Care,* Mosby, St. Louis, 1974.

Eisenstadt, S. N., *From Generation to Generation,* Free Press, New York, 1964.

Emery, F. E. (ed.), *Systems Thinking,* Penguin Books, Baltimore, 1974.

Etzioni, A., *Modern Organizations,* Prentice-Hall, Englewood Cliffs, New Jersey, 1964.

Griffiths, D. E., *Administrative Theory,* Prentice-Hall, Englewood Cliffs, New Jersey, 1959.

Gulich, L. H., *Papers on the Science of Administration,* Columbia University Press, New York, 1937.

Katz, D., and Kahn, R. L., *The Social Psychology of Organizations,* John Wiley & Sons, New York, 1966.

Kast, F., and Rosenzweig, J., *Organization and Management,* McGraw-Hill, New York, 1970.

Likert, R., *The Human Organization: Its Management and Value,* McGraw-Hill, New York, 1967.

Linton, R., *The Study of Man,* Appleton-Century-Crofts, New York, 1936.

McDonough, A. M., and Garrett, L. J., *Management Systems,* Irwin, Homewood, Illinois, 1965.

McGregor, D., McGregor, C., and Bennis, W. G. (eds.), *The Professional Manager,* McGraw-Hill, New York, 1976.

Massie, J. L., *Essentials of Management,* 2nd ed., Prentice-Hall, Englewood Cliffs, New Jersey, 1971.

Mayhew, B. E., Social Organization of Hospitals and Physicians, *Journal of Nursing Administration,* 1(5), September–October 1971, 25–31.

Milio, N., Health Care Organizations and Innovation, *Journal of Health and Social Behavior,* June 1971, 163–173.

Parsons, T., *The Social System,* Free Press, New York, 1964.

Peter, L. J., and Hull, R., *The Peter Principle,* Morrow, New York, 1969.

Raia, A. P., *Managing by Objectives,* Scott, Foresman, Glenview, Illinois, 1974.

Reddin, W. J., *Effective Management by Objectives,* McGraw-Hill, New York, 1971.

Simon, H. A., *Administrative Behavior,* 2nd ed. The Free Press, New York, 1965.

Smith, D., Organizational Theory and the Hospital, *Journal of Nursing Administration,* 2(3), May–June 1972, 19–23.

Taylor, F. W., *Scientific Management,* Harper & Row, New York, 1947.
Thompson, J. D., *Organization in Action,* McGraw-Hill, New York, 1967.
Townsend, R., *Up the Organization,* Fawcett, Greenwich, Connecticut, 1970.
Weber, M., *The Theory of Social and Economic Organization,* translated by A. M. Henderson and Talcott Parsons, Free Press, New York, 1947.

## AUTHORITY

Bates, F. L., and White, R. F., Differential Perceptions of Authority in Hospitals, *Journal of Health and Human Behavior,* 2, Winter 1961, 262-267.
Benne, K., *A Conception of Authority,* Russell and Russell, New York, 1971.
Bennis, W. G., Berkowitz, M., Affinito, M., and Malone, M., Authority, Power and the Ability to Influence, *Human Relations,* 11, May 1958, 143-155.
Blau, P. M., The Hierarchy of Authority in Organzations, *American Journal of Sociology,* 73, April 1967, 543-567.
Coser, R. L., Authority and Decision Making in a Hospital: A Comparative Analysis, *American Sociological Review,* 23, February 1958, 56-63.
Dalton, G. W., Barnes, L. B., and Zaleznik, A., *The Distribution of Authority in Formal Organizations,* Harvard University Press, Cambridge, Massachusetts, 1968.
DeGeorge, R. T., The Nature and Function of Epistemic Authority, in *Authority: A Philosophical Analysis,* edited by R. B. Harris, University of Alabama Press, Birmingham, Alabama, 1976.
Dornbusch, S. M., and Scott, R. W., *Evaluation and the Exercise of Authority,* Jossey-Bass, Belmont, California, 1975.
Gibson, J., Power vs. Authority: Fundamentals of Leadership, *The Clearing House,* November 1975, 116-118.
Gillam, R., Hierarchies in Nursing, *International Nursing Review,* 17, 1970, 312.
Goldstone, P., and Tunnell, D., A Critique of the Command Theory of Authority, *Educational Theory,* 24, Spring 1975, 131-138.
Guzzard, M. B., Sr., Acceptance of Authoritarianism in the Nurse by the Hospitalized Teenager, *Nursing Research,* 18(5), September-October 1969, 426.
Harris, R. B., (ed.), *Authority: A Philosophical Analysis,* University of Alabama Press, Birmingham, Alabama, 1976.
Hodgkinson, H., and Meeth, L. R., *Power and Authority,* Jossey-Bass, Belmont, California, 1971.
Kalisch, B., Of Half Gods and Mortals: Aesculapian Authority, *Nursing Outlook,* 23, January 1975, 22-28.
Lasswell, H. D., and Kaplan, A., *Power and Society: A Framework for Political Inquiry,* Yale University Press, New Haven, 1960.
Mahowald, J. F., Freeman, J. F., and Dietsche, B., Decentralization of Nursing Authority, *Supervisor Nurse,* March 1974, 40-46.
Manschreck, C. L. (ed.), *Erosion of Authority,* Abingdon Press, New York, 1971.

Meissner, W. W., *The Assault on Authority,* Orbis Books, New York, 1971.
O'Donnell, C. P. (ed.), *Freedom and Community,* Fordham University Press, New York, 1968.
Peabody, R. L., *Organizational Authority,* Atherton Press, New York, 1964.
Rogan, J., What Is Authority? *Nursing Mirror,* 134, January 28, 1972, 17-18.
Silk, D. N., Aspects of the Concept of Authority in Education, *Educatinal Theory,* 26, Summer 1976, 271-278.
Simon, Y. R., *A General Theory of Authority,* University of Notre Dame Press, South Bend, Indiana, 1962.

## POWER AND STATUS

Aiken, M., and Mott, F. (eds.), *Power Authority and Influence: The Structure of Community Power,* Random House, New York, 1970.
Arndt, C., and Huckaby, L., *Nursing Administration: Theory for Practice with a Systems Approach,* Mosby, St. Louis, 1980.
Ashley J., This I Believe about Power in Nursing, *Nursing Outlook,* 21(10), October 1973, 637-641.
Ashley, J., Power, Freedom and Professional Practice in Nursing, *Supervisor Nurse,* January 1975, 12-29.
Bandman, E., There Is Nothing Automatic about Rights, *American Journal of Nursing,* 77(5), May 1977, 867-872.
Berle, A. A., *Power,* Harcourt, New York, 1969.
Bowman, R. A., and Culpepper, R. C., Power, Rx for Change, *American Journal of Nursing,* 74,(6), June 1974, 1053-56.
Chaska, N. L., Status Consistency and Nurses' Expectations and Perceptions of Role Performance, *Nursing Research,* 27(6), November-December 1978, 356-364.
Claus, K. E., and Bailey, J. T., *Power and Influence in Health Care: A New Approach to Leadership,* Mosby, St. Louis, 1977.
Elsberry, N., Power Relations in Hospital Nursing, *Journal of Nursing Administration,* 2(5) September-October 1972, 75-77.
Etzioni, A. A., *Comparative Analysis of Complex Organizations,* Rev. Ed., Free Press, New York, 1975.
Glaser, B. G., and Strauss, A., *Status Passage,* Aldine, Chicago, 1971.
Jacobson, W. D., *Power and Interpersonal Relations,* Wadsworth, Belmont, California, 1972.
Kelly, D., Power and Its Abuse, *Supervisor Nurse,* November 1975, 7-8.
Korda, M., *Power: How to Get It How to Use It,* Random House, New York, 1975.
Laswell, H. D., and Kaplan, A., *Power and Society,* Yale University Press, New Haven, 1969.
Lieb, R., Power, Powerlessness and Potential—Nurse's Role within the Health Care Delivery System, *Image,* 10(3), October 1978. 75-82.

McClelland, D. C., *Power: The Inner Experience,* Irvington, New York, 1975.

McFarland, D. E., and Shiflett, N., The Role of Power in the Nursing Profession, *Nursing Dimensions,* 7(2), Summer 1979, 28–32.

Manthey, M., Ciske, K., Robertson, P., and Harris, I., Primary Nursing: A Return to the Concept of My Nurse and My Patient, *Nursing Forum,* 9(1), 1970, 64–83.

May, R., *Power and Innocence,* Norton, New York, 1972.

Miller, D. C., *International Community Power Structures,* Indiana University Press, Bloomington, 1970.

Moses, E., and Roth, A., Nursepower, *American Journal of Nursing,* 79(10), October 1979, 1745–1756.

Olsen, M. E., *Power in Societies,* Macmillan, New York, 1970.

Reilly, J. A., Power Persuasion, in *Quality Patient Care and the Role of the Clinical Nursing Specialist,* edited by R. Rotkovitch, John Wiley & Sons, New York, 1976.

Sampson, R., *The Psychology of Power,* Random House, New York, 1966.

Schorr, T., Nurse Power, *American Journal of Nursing,* 74(6), June 1974, 1047.

Smith, H. L., The Hospital's Dual Status System, in *Organizations and Human Behavior,* edited by G. Bell, Prentice-Hall, Englewood Cliffs, New Jersey, 1967, pp. 109–117.

Swingle, P.G., *The Management of Power,* John Wiley & Sons, New York, 1976.

Zald, M. N. (ed.), *Power in Organization,* Vanderbilt University Press, Nashville, Tennessee, 1970.

Zaleznick, A., Power and Accountability, in *Management for Nurses: A Multidisciplinary Approach,* edited by S. Stone, et al., Mosby, St. Louis, 1976, pp. 13–33.

# DECISION MAKING

Baker, F., (ed.), *Organizational Systems: General Systems Approaches to Complex Organizations,* Irwin, Homewood, Illinois, 1973.

Barnard, C. I., *The Functions of the Executive,* Macmillan, New York, 1954.

Beer, S., *Decision and Control,* John Wiley & Sons, New York, 1966.

Bross, I., *Design for Decision,* Macmillan, New York, 1953.

Drucker, P. F., *The Effective Executive,* Harper & Row, New York, 1967.

Grier, M. R., Decision Making about Patient Care, *Nursing Research,* 76(2), March–April 1976, 105–110.

Griffiths, D., *Administrative Theory,* Prentice-Hall, Englewood Cliffs, New Jersey, 1959.

Hansen, A. C., and Thomas, D. B., A Conceptualization of Decision Making, *Nursing Research,* 17(5), September–October 1968, 536–543.

Hansen, A. C., Differences and Changes in Decision Judgments within Two Role Groups, *Nursing Research,* 18(4), July–August 1969, 333–338.

Hansen, A. C., Professionalization of Priority Decision Judgments, *Nursing Research,* 19(4), July–August 1970, 343–348.

Hiscoe, S., The Awesome Decision, *American Journal of Nursing,* 73(2), February 1973, 291-293.

Johnson, B. M., Decision Making, Faculty Satisfaction and the Place of Nursing in the University, *Nursing Research,* 22(2), March-April 1973, 100-107.

Kast, F. E., and Rosenweig, J. E., *Organization and Management: A Systems Approach,* McGraw-Hill, New York, 1974.

Kelley, K., Clinical Inference in Nursing, *Nursing Research,* 15(1), Winter 1966, 23-26.

Kolb, D. A., Rubin, I. M., and McIntyre, J. (eds.), *Organizational Psychology—A Book of Readings,* 2nd ed., Prentice-Hall, Englewood Cliffs, New Jersey, 1974.

LaMonica, E., and Finch, F. E., Managerial Decision Making, *Journal of Nursing Administration,* 7(5), May-June 1977, 20-28.

Miller, D. W., and Starr, M. K., *The Structure of Human Decisions,* Prentice-Hall, Englewood Cliffs, New Jersey, 1967.

Olson, M., Social Influence on Decision Making, *Journal of Nursing Education,* 7(1), January 1968, 11-16.

Peter, L. U., *The Peter Prescription,* Morrow, New York, 1972.

Schaefer, J., The Interrelatedness of Decision Making and the Nursing Process, *American Journal of Nursing,* 74(10), October 1974, 1852-1855.

Simon, H. A., *Administrative Behavior,* 2nd ed. Macmillan, New York, 1957.

Smiley, O. R., The Core Committee . . . A Model for Decision Making within Public Health Units, *Nursing Clinics of North America,* 8(2), June 1973, 355-359.

Sumidal, S. W., A Computerized Test for Clinical Decision Making, *Nursing Outlook,* 20, July 1972, 458-461.

Thomas, D. B., and Hansen, A. C., Multiple Discriminant Analysis of Public Health Nursing Decision Responses, *Nursing Research,* 18(2), March-April 1969, 145-153.

Young, J., A Conceptual Framework for Hospital Administrative Decision Systems, *Health Services Research,* Summer 1968, 79-95.

# 5
# A Theory of Goal Attainment

Three dynamic interacting systems have been presented as an open systems framework for nursing. Since systems have goals, a concept of health was developed that described the goals for nursing. This framework can be summarized as follows:

> Individuals comprise one type of system in the environment called personal systems. Individuals interact to form dyads, triads, and small and large groups, which comprise another type of system called interpersonal systems. Groups with special interests and needs form organizations, which make up communities and societies and are called social systems.

The abstract concepts are human beings, environment, health, and society. These concepts help nurses gain special knowledge of human beings and environment and some of the critical variables that influence behavior. Knowledge of these concepts helps nurses understand that through human interactions, based on perceptions, human beings perform activities of daily living in various roles in social systems. Adjustments to life and health are influenced by individual's interactions with environment.

A major thesis of the framework is that each human being perceives the world as a total person in making transactions with individuals and things in the environment. Perceiving takes place in each person's concrete world and is an essential part of living. Transactions represent a life situation in which perceiver and thing perceived are encountered and in which each person enters the situation as an active participant, and each is changed in the process of these experiences.

Major concepts identified within each of the three interacting systems were developed as substantive content for nursing. These concepts represent different levels of abstraction. For example, self is a higher level of abstraction than body image, yet they are related concepts.

A concept of self emerges in the process of growth and development through the life span, which is influenced by time and space. A concept of self influences one's perceptions, and one's perceptions help develop a concept of self. If this sounds circular, it is, because they are facets of human experience.

Perception, self, growth and development, time, and space influence role conception, role taking, role expectations, and role performance. Knowledge of these concepts helps nurses begin to understand self and the behaviors of other individuals. Knowledge is used as nurses interact with clients in a variety of health care systems. In the process of interaction, nurses and clients are sharing information through communication, and are making transactions in the situations to meet their goals. When the goals of the nurse and the goals of the client are incongruent, conflict may occur and increase stress in both individuals and in the situation.

The delivery of quality care in health care systems is expected by the public. One measure of quality is a measure of effectiveness of care. Effectiveness of care can be measured by whether or not the goals for health promotion, health maintenance, or recovery from illness have been attained.

A theory of goal attainment has been derived from this open systems framework. Although personal systems and social systems influence quality of care, the major elements in a theory of goal attainment are discovered in the interpersonal systems in which two people, who are usually strangers, come together in a health care organization to help and to be helped to maintain a state of health that permits functioning in roles.

This theory describes the nature of nurse–client interactions that lead to achievement of goals. It presents a standard for nurse–patient interactions, namely, that nurses purposefully interact with clients mutually to establish goals and to explore and agree on means to achieve goals. Mutual goal setting is based on nurses' assessment of client's concerns, problems, and disturbances in health, their perceptions of problems, and their sharing information to move toward goal attainment. This theory, derived from the conceptual framework, organizes elements in the process of nurse-client interactions that result in outcomes, that is, goals attained.

It is possible that other theories could be derived from this open systems framework. For example, interpersonal stress theory, control theory, or a general theory of human behavior may be considered. Before explication of the theory, specific assumptions are presented.

## Philosophical Assumptions

The conceptual framework and the theory of goal attainment are based on an overall assumption that the focus of nursing is human beings interacting with their environment leading to a state of health for individuals, which is an ability to function in social roles. Specific assumptions about human beings are:

- Individuals are social beings.
- Individuals are sentient beings.
- Individuals are rational beings.
- Individuals are reacting beings.
- Individuals are perceiving beings.
- Individuals are controlling beings.
- Individuals are purposeful beings.
- Individuals are action-oriented beings.
- Individuals are time-oriented beings.

Specific assumptions about nurse-client interactions are:

- Perceptions of nurse and of client influence the interaction process.
- Goals, needs, and values of nurse and client influence the interaction process.
- Individuals have a right to knowledge about themselves.
- Individuals have a right to participate in decisions that influence their life, their health, and community services.
- Health professionals have a responsibility to share information that helps individuals make informed decisions about their health care.
- Individuals have a right to accept or to reject health care.

- Goals of health professionals and goals of recipients of health care may be incongruent.

A personal philosophy of human beings influenced the development of the conceptual framework and the theory of goal attainment.

## Major Concepts in the Theory

Theory is defined as a set of interrelated concepts, definitions, and propositions that present a systematic view of essential elements in a field of inquiry by specifying relations among variables (Nagel, 1961; Kerlinger, 1973; Fawcett, 1978).

A theory of goal attainment was derived from the conceptual framework of interpersonal systems. The dyad, nurse and client, is one type of interpersonal system. The theory utilized concepts of interaction, perception, communication, transaction, role, stress, growth and development. It is postulated that nurse and client interactions are characterized by verbal and nonverbal communication, in which information is exchanged and interpreted; by transactions, in which values, needs, and wants of each member of the dyad are shared; by perceptions of nurse and client and the situation; by self in role of client and self in role of nurse; and by stressors influencing each person and the situation in time and space.

In constructing a theory of goal attainment, a definition of nursing was formulated. Nursing is a process of human interactions between nurse and client whereby each perceives the other and the situation; and through communication, they set goals, explore means, and agree on means to achieve goals. For example, one goal may be to help a client learn how to cope with a chronic illness. Another example may be to help a patient regain the use of a right hand. This definition implies that actions and reactions take place in each nursing situation. The behaviors that are observable in nurse and client are: (1) recognition of presenting conditions, such as a health problem, a social problem, or a human concern; (2) operations or activities related to the situation or conditions, such as decisions about goals; (3) motivation to exert some control over the events in the situation to achieve goals, such as agreement on means to achieve them. Within these interactions nurses gather information, observe and measure parameters of clients, interpret the information, give appropriate information to the client to help set goals; clients observe the nurse, ask questions, give information, and participate in setting goals. Goals are perceived as events that one values, wants, or desires. Goal attainment results in outcomes that are measurable events in nursing situations. This theory should serve as a standard of practice related to nurse–patient interactions, and is in this sense a normative theory.

## DEFINITION OF THE CONCEPTS

The major concepts in the theory of goal attainment are interaction, perception, communication, transaction, self, role, stress, growth and development, and time and space.

**Interaction.** This concept is defined as a process of perception and communication between person and environment and between person and person, represented by verbal and nonverbal behaviors that are goal-directed. In person-to-person interactions, each individual brings different knowledge, needs, goals, past experiences, and perceptions, which influence the interactions. A human interaction diagram showing nurse and client interactions is seen in Figure 5.1. It is identical to Figure 3.1 but with specific individuals in role (King, 1971). When two individuals come together for a purpose, such as in a nursing situation, they are each perceiving the other person and the situation, making judgments, taking mental action, or making a decision to act. These two individuals react

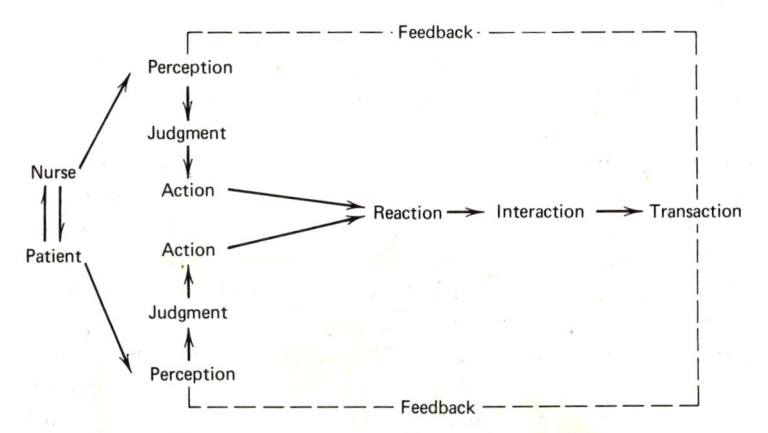

**Figure 5.1** A process of human interactions.

Reprinted with permission from I. M. King, *Toward a Theory for Nursing*, New York, John Wiley & Sons, 1971, p. 92.

to each other and the situation. All of these behaviors are not directly observable. Inferences are made about what each is perceiving and thinking. Accuracy in perception will depend upon verifying one's inferences with the client. Interactions are directly observable behaviors whereby a trained observer can record verbal and nonverbal behaviors of nurse and client as they interact. The raw data of these interactions, not the inferences of nurses, can be analyzed to identify transactions made.

**Perception.** Perception is defined as each person's representation of reality. It is an awareness of persons, objects, and events. Perception involves the following elements: (1) import of energy from the environment organized by information, (2) transformation of energy, (3) processing of information, (4) storing of information, (5) export of information in overt behaviors. One's perceptions are related to past experiences, concept of self, socioeconomic groups, biological inheritance, and educational background. A useful definition of the perceptual process is:

> ... perceiving refers to the process by which a particular person from his particular behavioral center attributes significance to his immediate environmental situation. And the significances which he attributes are those which he discovered from past experiences have furthered his purposes.... While present and past are involved in the perceptual process, the chief time orientation in perceiving is toward the future. (Ittleson and Cantril, 1954, pp. 26–27)

Perception is each person's subjective world of experience.

**Communication.** Communication is defined as a process whereby information is given from one person to another either directly in face-to-face meetings or indirectly through telephone, television, or the written word. Communication is the information component of the interactions. Information is communicated in a variety of ways between nurses and clients, nurses and families, and nurses and physicians and allied professionals. Communication establishes a mutuality between care givers and recipients of care. Communication is the means by which information is given in specific nursing situations to identify concerns and/or problems, to share information that assists individuals in making decisions that lead to goal attainment in the environment. Human behavior that relates person to person and person to environment is communication. The means used to share information and ideas are verbal and nonverbal signs and symbols by which individuals also express their goals.

**Transaction.** Transaction is defined as observable behavior of human beings interacting with their environment. Transactions are viewed as the valuation component of human interactions. If nurses and clients make transactions in nursing situations, they communicate in order to exchange their values relative to the situation. This involves bargaining, negotiating, and social exchange. When nurses and clients share their frame of reference about events in the present, they identify commonalities whereby they can mutually set goals. When transactions are made between nurses and clients, goals are attained. Role expectations and role performance of nurses and clients influence transactions.

**Role.** Role is defined as a set of behaviors expected of persons occupying a position in a social system; rules that define rights and obligations in a position; a relationship with one or more individuals interacting in specific situations for a purpose. Role of a nurse is defined by the functions expected of professional nurses based on knowledge, skills, and values of the profession. Those functions are identified in nursing process as assessment of clients, using the information to plan for goal setting, implementing means to achieve goal, and evaluating whether or not goal is attained. If expectations of employers differ from expectations of nurses, role conflict may exist. The dilemma is that employers have one set of expectations, allied health professionals have another set of expectations, and clients have yet another set of expectations. It is important for nurses to understand and interpret their role to others. Role conflict and role confusion decrease achievement of effective care for clients and create stress in situations.

**Stress.** Stress is defined as a dynamic state whereby a human being interacts with the environment to maintain balance for growth, development, and performance. This involves an exchange of energy and information between the person and the environment for regulation and control of stressors. Stress is an energy response of an individual to persons, objects, and events called stressors. Nurses are expected to decrease stressors in the hospital for patients and families, yet few support systems are offered to reduce stressors for nurses. One of the stressors in hospital nursing is the constantly changing working hours from days to evenings and to nights. This constant change interferes with nurses' biological rhythms. One of the stressors in patients' environments is sensory deprivation; another is sensory overload. When stress is increased in the individuals interacting in a situation, their perceptual field narrows and their decision making decreases in rationality. These factors may lead to decreased interactions and goal setting and to ineffective nursing care. In addition, interference in each person's developmental tasks may occur.

**Growth and development.** These concepts are defined as continuous changes in individuals at the cellular, molecular, and behavioral levels of activities. Growth and development are a function of genetic endowment, meaningful and satisfying experiences, and an environment conducive to helping individuals move toward maturity. Growth and development have been defined as the processes that take place in the life of individuals that help them move from potential capacity for achievement to self-actualization. Age is a critical variable that defines this movement and the stage of each person's developmental tasks. Age implies time.

**Time.** Time is defined as a sequence of events moving onward to the future. Time is a continuous flow of events in successive order that implies change, a past, and a future. Time is a duration between one event and another as uniquely experienced by each human being; it is the relation of one event to another. Time is related to rhythmicity in the functions of human beings and can be seen in fluctuations in body temperature, elimination of waste products, sleep and wake cycles, metabolism, and fluid and electrolyte balance. Changes in work hours may disrupt nurses' body rhythms. Time perceptions of patients in hospitals are important in nurse–patient interactions. Interactions in hospitals take place in particular places, such as patients' rooms, which restrict space.

**Space.** Space is defined as existing in all directions and is the same everywhere. Space is a physical area called territory, and is defined by the behavior of individuals occupying space, such as gestures, postures, and visible boundaries erected to mark off personal space. The use of space communicates messages with different meanings in different cultures. The perception of space will influence the way individuals behave in certain situations. Limited space for patients and nurses in critical care units in hospitals may influence their behaviors. Spatial distance and closeness are factors to consider in nurse–client interactions. Space is explicit in this theory because it is the immediate environment in which nurse and client interact and move to goal attainment.

The concepts in the theory have been defined and propositions that link these concepts are presented.

## Propositions

According to Dubin (1978) a proposition is a truth statement about a theory. Propositions give consideration to the function of a theory as a dynamic system. Some of the following propositions deal with process and others with outcomes:

1. If perceptual accuracy is present in nurse–client interactions, transactions will occur.
2. If nurse and client make transactions, goals will be attained.
3. If goals are attained, satisfactions will occur.
4. If goals are attained, effective nursing care will occur.
5. If transactions are made in nurse–client interactions, growth and development will be enhanced.
6. If role expectations and role performance as perceived by nurse and client are congruent, transactions will occur.
7. If role conflict is experienced by nurse or client or both, stress in nurse–client interactions will occur.
8. If nurses with special knowledge and skills communicate appropriate information to clients, mutual goal setting and goal attainment will occur.

The above propositions give some idea of the predictive value of the concepts in the theory. Additional propositions may be generated from the theory.

## Boundaries of the Theory

If a theory is to represent an empirical system, its boundaries must correspond to the empirical system. The theoretical formulations are concerned with the analysis of nurse–client interactions that lead to goal attainment in natural environments.

Interior boundary determining criteria are:

1. Nurse and client do not know each other.
2. Nurse is licensed to practice professional nursing.
3. Client is in need of the services provided by the nurse.
4. Nurse and client are in a reciprocal relationship in that the nurse has special knowledge and skills to communicate appropriate information to help client set goals; client has information about self and perceptions of problems or concerns that when communicated to nurse will help in mutual goal setting.
5. Nurse and client are in mutual presence, purposefully interacting to achieve goals.

According to Dubin (1978), interior criteria are derived from the characteristics of the concepts and are internal to the theory.

Exterior boundary criteria are: (1) interactions in a two-person group; (2) interactions limited to licensed professional nurse and to client in need of nursing care; (3) interactions taking place in natural environments. The boundaries of a theory define the domain of the theory (Dubin, 1978). These boundaries do not restrict the theory to time and place, as nurse–client interactions can occur in any nursing situation at any time and in any place. If a theory is to be useful, it must be tested.

## Testing the Theory

Numerous studies and reports about the importance of communication, interaction, and interpersonal relations for nursing practice have appeared in the nursing literature. These ideas were useful in developing the theory of goal attainment.

Before designing a descriptive study to explain nurse–client interactions that lead to transactions, an operational definition of transaction had to be developed. Continuous time series data of observations of nurse–patient interactions in one hospital were available, from which a definition of transaction was inductively developed. This definition identified a transaction in the hospital setting as follows:

1. One member of the nurse–patient dyad initiates behavior; asks question; makes statement; reaches out with arms; walks toward other; looks at the other; gives something to other.

2. Opposite member of the nurse-patient dyad responds with behavior; answers question; makes statement; reaches out with arms; walks toward other; returns look; gives or accepts something from other.
3. Disturbance (or problem) is noted in the dyadic situation if a state or condition is identified: for example, intravenous infusion is all right or is infiltrating; pain is stated by one member, or perceived by another member; procedure is carried out or refused; resistance to act related to patient condition; activities related to patient state are recognized and performed, or not.
4. Some goal is mutually agreed upon by members of dyad; goal may be implicit in behavior that is observed or verbalized; each member shows or states agreement.
5. Exploration of means to achieve goals is initiated by one member of dyad, or behavior is exhibited by member of dyad that moves toward goal: for example, preoperative teaching of deep breathing and coughing to help the postoperative recovery period; plan to exercise hand and arm to prevent contractures; teaching mother how to protect child's burns to promote healing.
6. Other member agrees with means to achieve goal; both move toward goal.
7. Transactions are made; goal is attained.

The first phase of testing the theory was to describe nurse-patient interactions that lead to transactions in concrete nursing situations. A study* was designed to answer three questions:

1. What elements in nurse-patient interactions lead to transactions?
2. What are the relationships between the elements in the interactions that lead to transactions?
3. What are the essential variables in nurse-patient interactions that result in transactions?

This study described an interpersonal system of nurse-patient interactions. A major assumption in the study was that the nurse and the patient exhibit reciprocally interactive behavior; that is, the behavior of one person influences the behavior of the other person and vice versa.
Several theoretical formulations about interpersonal relations and

---

*Partially supported by Loyola University of Chicago.

nursing process have been described in nursing situations (Peplau, 1952; Orlando, 1961; King, 1971; Paterson and Zderad, 1977; Yura and Walsh, 1978). Few nursing studies have provided empirical data about nursing process phenomena related to human interaction.

## BACKGROUND

Ideas about a human process of interaction served as a framework for beginning to describe systematically nurse-patient interactions in concrete nursing situations. Knowledge of perception is essential for nurses to understand interactions. Perception can be studied only in terms of the transactions in which the facts of perception can be observed (Ittleson and Cantril, 1954).

Transaction, another important concept in this theory, has been reported in a theory of knowledge (Dewey and Bentley, 1949) and in studies of perception and studies of thinking (Allport, 1955; Laing, Phillipson, and Lee, 1966; Bruner, 1956). Kuhn (1975) noted that transactions are the valuational component in human interactions and that communications are the informational component. Verbal and nonverbal behaviors recorded in this study demonstrated informational components of interactions. When a goal is achieved in nurse-patient interactions, there is an implication that it was valued by nurse and patient.

Theories of interpersonal perception and interpersonal relations provided some theoretical background for using a human process of interaction to describe and classify nurse-patient interactions. A dual system for classifying interactions that deal with variations in situations was proposed: (1) in terms of reciprocity of behavior from one extreme of mutual dependent behavior to the other extreme of mutual independent behavior, and (2) in terms of mediated goals (Jones and Thibaut, 1958). In a nursing situation, one can observe reciprocally contingent interactions in which the behavior of the patient is contingent on the behavior of the nurse and vice versa. In addition, nurses and patients communicate information to each other to achieve mutual goals.

Orlando's study of a deliberative nursing process noted the importance of nurses' and patients' perceptions and their influence on interactions. Her findings support the idea that nursing process is reciprocal and that nurses and patients identify goals (Orlando, 1972).

A descriptive study was conducted to begin to test this theory of goal attainment. The purpose of the study was to analyze data from nurse-patient interactions to search for transactions in concrete nursing situa-

```
                        Action

         ELEMENTS IN INTERACTIONS
                        Reaction

                        Disturbance

                        Mutual goal setting

                        Explore means to achieve goal

                        Agree on means to achieve goal

                        Transaction — goal achieved
```

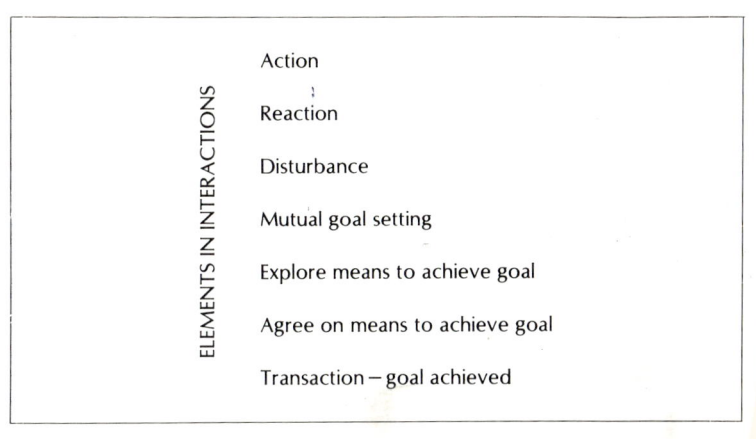

**Figure 5.2** Classification system of nurse–patient interactions.

phase in testing this theory is to design experimental studies to test hypotheses generated from the theory.

## Hypotheses

The following hypotheses are derived from the theory:

1. Perceptual accuracy in nurse–patient interactions increases mutual goal setting.
2. Communication increases mutual goal setting between nurses and patients and leads to satisfactions.
3. Satisfactions in nurses and patients increase goal attainment.
4. Goal attainment decreases stress and anxiety in nursing situations.
5. Goal attainment increases patient learning and coping ability in nursing situations.
6. Role conflict experienced by patients, nurses, or both, decreases transactions in nurse–patient interactions.
7. Congruence in role expectations and role performance increases transactions in nurse–patient interactions.

One approach to help nurses study the complexity of nursing has been demonstrated in the initial testing of a theory of goal attainment. The

Table 5.1. **Frequencies and Percentages of Interactions that Lead to Transactions**

| Categories | | No Transactions | Transactions |
|---|---|---|---|
| Actions | | 5 | 12 |
| | | 29.4% | 70.6% |
| Reactions | | 5 | 12 |
| | | 29.4% | 70.6% |
| Disturbances | | 5 | 12 |
| | | 29.4% | 70.6% |
| Goals explored | No | 3 | 0 |
| | | 17.6% | 0.0% |
| | Yes | 2 | 12 |
| | | 11.8% | 70.6% |
| Explore means to achieve goal(s) | No | 4 | 0 |
| | | 23.5% | 0.% |
| | Yes | 1 | 12 |
| | | 5.9% | 70.6% |
| Agree to means to achieve goal(s) | No | 4 | 0 |
| | | 23.5% | 0.0% |
| | Yes | 1 | 12 |
| | | 5.9% | 70.6% |

$N$ = 17 nurse-patient interactions.

The third question was: what are the essential variables in nurse-patient interactions that result in transactions? Variables that facilitated goal attainment were accurate perceptions of nurse and patient; adequate communication; mutual goal setting.

This descriptive study resulted in a classification system to analyze nurse-patient interactions as shown in Figure 5.2. A schematic diagram in Figure 5.3 shows the process and the concepts in a relationship.

From this testing of a theory of goal attainment at a descriptive level, a classification system was designed, and the theory is useful in nursing. The theory focuses on goals to be attained in specific nursing situations through participative decision making by nurses and patients. If nurses and the future students in nursing were taught this theory of goal attainment and used it in nursing situations, accurate recording of goals identified and goals attained in nurse-patient interactions could be documented, and effectiveness of nursing care could be measured. The next

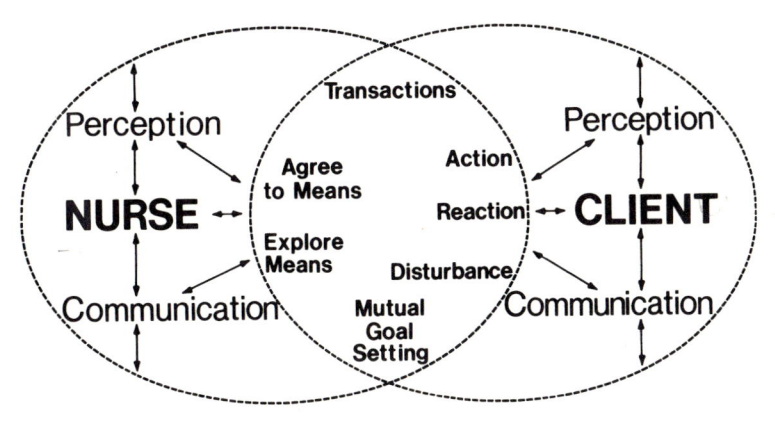

**Figure 5.3** Schematic diagram of a theory of goal attainment.

theory was derived from the conceptual framework of dynamic interacting systems, especially interpersonal systems.

## Summary

A useful theory is hard to invent without some description of the empirical world of nursing. Theory construction and hypotheses testing is a time-consuming activity. Theory, because it is abstract, cannot be immediately applied to nursing practice or to concrete nursing education programs. When empirical referents are identified, defined, and described, as in this chapter, theory is useful and can be applied in concrete situations.

There is a basic assumption in the theory presented, that is, that generally patients and nurses communicate information, mutually set goals, and take action to attain goals. Some of the essential variables have been identified in the empirical description of the theory of goal attainment that provides knowledge of process and outcomes. Process and outcomes are the heart of quality assurance programs in nursing. The theory of goal attainment can be used by nurses. A Goal Oriented Nursing Record (modified from ideas of the Problem Oriented Medical Record) will facilitate the application of this theory in health care systems. This type of nursing record is discussed in the next chapter.

# Bibliography

## GOAL ATTAINMENT

Allport, F., *Theories of Perception and the Concept of Structure*, John Wiley & Sons, New York, 1955.

Anderson, M.D., Human Interaction for Nurses, *Supervisor Nurse*, 44, October 1979, 48–50.

Bennis, W. G., Berlew, D. E., Schein, E. H., and Steele, F. I., *Interpersonal Dynamics: Essays and Readings in Human Interaction*, Dorsey Press, Homewood, Illinois, 1976.

Bruner, J., *The Process of Education*, Harvard University Press, Cambridge, Massachusetts, 1960.

Bruner, J., Goodnow, J., and Austin, G., *A Study of Thinking*, John Wiley & Sons, New York, 1956.

Daubenmire, M. J., and King, I. M., Nursing Process Models: A Systems Approach, *Nursing Outlook*, 21, August 1973, 512–517.

Dewey, J., *The Quest for Certainty: A Study of the Relation between Knowledge and Action*, Putnam's, New York, 1960.

Dewey, J., and Bentley, A., *Knowing and the Known*, Beacon Press, Boston, 1949.

Dewey, J., and Bentley, A., Knowing and the Known, in *Useful Procedures of Inquiry*, edited by R. Bandy and E. C. Harwood, Behavior Research Council, Great Barrington, Massachusetts, 1973, 9–13.

Diers, D., and Schmidt, F. Interaction Analysis in Nursing Research, in *Nursing Research II*, edited by P. Varhonick, Little, Brown, Boston, 1977.

Dubin, R., *Theory Building*, rev. ed., Free Press, New York, 1978.

Egan, G., *Interpersonal Living*, Brooks/Cole, Monterey, California, 1976.

Fawcett, J., The What of Theory Development, in *Theory Development: What, Why, How*, National League for Nursing, New York, 1978, pp. 17–33.

Howland, D., Models in Nursing Research, in *Nursing Research II*, edited by P. Verhonick, Little, Brown, Boston, 1977, 135–148.

Ittleson, W., and Cantril, H., *Perception—A Transactional Approach*, Doubleday, Garden City, New York, 1954.

Jones, E. E., and Thibaut, J. W., Interaction Goals as Bases of Interference in Interpersonal Perception, in *Personal Perception and Interpersonal Behavior*, edited by R. Tagiuri and L. Petrullo, Stanford University Press, Palo Alto, California, 1958, 151–178.

Kelley, H., and Thibaut, J., *Interpersonal Relations: A Theory of Interdependence*, John Wiley & Sons, New York, 1978.

Kerlinger, F., *Foundations of Behavioral Reserach*, 2nd ed. Holt, Rinehart & Winston, New York, 1973.

King, I. M., *Toward a Theory for Nursing*, John Wiley & Sons, New York, 1971.

King, I. M., A. Process for Developing Concepts for Nursing Research, in *Nursing Research II,* edited by P. Verhonick, Little, Brown, Boston, 1975, 25-44.

King, I. M., The Decision Maker's Perspective: Patient Care Aspects, in *Operations Research in Health Care: A Critical Analysis,* edited by L. Schuman, R. Dixon Speas, and J. P. Young, Johns Hopkins Press, Baltimore, 1975, 3-20.

King, I. M., Reaction letter to George Annas and Joseph Healy article entitled "The Patient Rights Advocate," *The Journal of Nursing Administration,* Vol. 5(1), 1975, 40-41.

King, I. M., Health Care Systems: Nursing Intervention Subsystems, In *Health Research: The Systems Approach,* edited by H. Werley, et al., Springer Publishing Co., New York, 1976, 51-60.

King, I. M., The Why of Theory Development, in *Theory Development What, Why and How,* National League for Nursing, New York, 1978, 11-16.

King, I. M., *Nursing Theory,* Audio tapes, Nursing Resources Inc., Wakefield, Massachusetts, 1978.

Kuhn, A., *Unified Social Science,* Dorsey Press, Homewood, Illinois, 1975.

Laing, R. D., Phillipson, H., and Lee, A. R., *Interpersonal Perception: A Theory and a Method of Research,* Harper & Row, New York, 1966.

Larson, P. Sr., Nurse Perceptions of Patient Characteristics, *Nursing Research,* Vol. 26(6), November-December 1977, 416-421.

Murray, J. E., Patient Participation in Determining Psychiatric Treatment, *Nursing Research,* Vol 23(4), July-August 1975, 325-333.

Orlando, I. J., *The Dynamic Nurse-Patient Relationship,* Putnam's, New York, 1961.

Orlando, I. J., *The Discipline and Teaching of Nursing Process,* Putnam's, New York, 1972.

Paterson, J., and Zderad, L., *Humanistic Nursing,* John Wiley & Sons, New York, 1976.

Peplau, H. *Interpersonal Relations in Nursing,* Putnam's, New York, 1952.

Rogers, C. R., *On Becoming a Person,* Houghton Mifflin, Boston, 1961.

Spiegel, J., *Transactions: The Interplay between Individual, Family and Society,* Science House, New York, 1971.

Taguiri, R., and Petrullo, L. (eds.), *Person Perception and Interpersonal Behavior,* Stanford University Press, Palo Alto, California, 1958.

Torres, G., and Yura, H., *Today's Conceptual Framework: Its Relationship to Curriculum Development Process,* National League for Nursing, New York, 1974.

Whiting, J. F., Q-Sort Technique for Evaluating Perceptions of Interpersonal Relationships, *Nursing Research,* 4, 1955, 71.

Whiting, J. F., Patients' Needs, Nurses' Needs and the Healing Process, *American Journal of Nursing,* 59(5), May 1959, 663.

Yura, H., and Walsh, M., *The Nursing Process,* Appleton-Century-Crofts, New York, 1978.

Zimmerman, D., and Gohrke, C. The Goal Directed Nursing, *American Journal of Nursing,* 70(2), February 1970, 306-310.

## GOAL-ORIENTED NURSING RECORD

American Nurses' Association, *Standards of Nursing Practice,* American Nurses' Association, Kansas City, 1973.

American Nurses' Association, *A Plan for Implementation of the Standards of Nursing Practice,* American Nurses' Association, Kansas City, 1975.

American Nurses' Association, *Guidelines for Review of Nursing Care at the Local Level,* American Nurses' Association, Kansas City, 1976.

Assessing the Quality of Care, *Nursing Outlook,* 23, March 1975, 153-159.

Barba, M. Bennett, B., and Shaw, W. J., The Evaluation of Patient Care through Use of ANA's Standards of Nursing Practice, *Supervisor Nurse,* January 1978, 52-54.

Berg, H. V., Nursing Audit and Outcome Criteria, *Nursing Clinics of North America,* 9(2), June 1974, 331-335.

Bertucci, M., Huston, M., and Perloff, E., Comparative Study of Progress Notes Using POMR and Traditional Methods of Charting, *Nursing Research,* 23(4), July-August 1974, 351-354.

Block, D., Evaluation of Nursing Care in Terms of Process and Outcome: Issues in Research and Quality Assurance, *Nursing Research,* 24(4), July-August 1975, 256-263.

Bonkowsky, M. L., Adapting the POMR to Community Child Health Care, *Nursing Outlook,* 20(8), August 1972, 515-518.

Deets, C., and Schmidt, A., Outcome Criteria Based on Standards, *AORN Journal,* 26(2), February 1978, 220-226.

Given, B., Given, C. W., Simmons, S., and Lewis, E., Relationships of Processes of Care to Patient Outcomes, *Nursing Research,* 28(2), March-April 1979, 85-93.

Hofing, A. L., McGugin, M. B., and Merkel, S. I., The Importance of Maintenance in Implementing Change: An Experience with Problem Oriented Recording, *The Journal of Nursing Administration,* 9, December 1979, 43-48.

Hover, J., and Zimmer, J. J., Nursing Quality Assurance: The Wisconsin System, *Nursing Outlook,* 26(4), April 1978, 242-248.

Jenny, J., A Humanistic Strategy for Patient Teaching, *Health Values: Achieving High Level Wellness,* 3(3), May-June 1979, 175-180.

McClure, M. K., Quality Assurance and Nursing Education: A Nursing Service Director's View, *Nursing Outlook,* 24(8), June 1976, 367-369.

Mayers, M. G., Norby, R. B., and Watson, A. B., *Quality Assurance for Patient Care: Nursing Perspectives,* Appleton-Century-Crofts, New York, 1977.

Mitchell, P., and Atwood, J., Problem Oriented Recording as a Teaching-Learning Tool, *Nursing Research,* 24(2), March-April 1975, 99-103.

Moore, K. R., What Nurses Learn from Nursing Audit, *Nursing Outlook,* 27(4), April 1979, 254-258.

Nagel, E., The Structure of Science, Harcourt, New York, 1961.

Nicholls, M. E., Quality Control in Patient Care, *American Journal of Nursing,* 74(3), March 1974, 456-459.

Nicholls, M. E., and Wessells, V. G. (eds.), *Nursing Standards and Nursing Process*, Contemporary Publishing, Wakefield, Massachusetts, 1977.

*Nursing Clinics of North America*, Symposium on Problem Oriented Record, Saunders, Philadelphia, 9(2), June 1974, 215–302.

*Nursing Clinics of North America*, Symposium on Quality Assurance, Saunders, Philadephia, 9(2), June 1974, 303–379.

Phaneuf, M. C., *The Nursing Audit: Self-Regulation in Nursing Practice*, Appleton-Century-Crofts, New York, 1976.

Schell, P. L., and Campbell, A. T., POMR-Not Just Another Way to Chart, *Nursing Outlook*, 20(8), August 1972, 510–514.

Schmadl, J. C., Quality Assurance: Examination of the Concept, *Nursing Outlook*, 27(7), July 1979, 462–465.

Slavitt, D. B., et al., Nurses' Satisfaction with Their Work Situation, *Nursing Research*, 27(2), March–April 1978, 114–120.

Walter, J. B., Pardee, G. P., and Molbo, D. M. (eds.), *Dynamics of Problem-Oriented Approaches: Patient Care and Documentation*, Lippincott, Philadelphia, 1976.

Woody, M., and Mallison, M., The Problem-Oriented System for Patient-Centered Care, *American Journal of Nursing*, 73(7), July 1973, 1168–1175.

# 6
# Application of a Theory of Goal Attainment in Nursing

Health care delivery for the future mandates an approach that promotes communication, cooperation, and coordination among health care providers. Nurses and physicians are two groups of major providers of health care in the United States. Coordination of a plan of care will occur if professionals recognize a common goal for recipients of care. That goal is to help individuals maintain a healthy state so they can function in society. The means to achieve a common goal vary with each professional group and its roles and functions in society.

The overall goal of physicians has been to diagnose, treat, and cure disease and illness. The overall goal of nurses has been to promote health, prevent disease, and care for the ill, injured, or dying. If communication and cooperation are to be achieved, each group must have some understanding of the functions, roles, relationships, and goals of the other group. In this way, both groups can understand distinct functions and relationships, and distinguish where there is some overlap in functions, as in patient education.

Over a decade ago, Dr. Weed (1969) recommended that physicians begin to use a logical way to document medical care. He designed a Problem-Oriented Medical Record, and this has been used by physicians who teach medical students, and by physicians in private practice and in community agencies (Bjorn and Cross, 1970; Hurst, 1972; Aradine and Guthneck, 1974). This record provides a logical, efficient, and effective method for recording patient problems and the actions taken to resolve them. In some institutions, nurses and other health professionals have adapted records of a similar nature or have used the Problem-Oriented Medical Record to document the care given. Some hospitals have initiated a separate nursing data base record system that is a modification of the Weed system (Woody and Mallison, 1973; Blount, et al., 1978; Hofing, et al., 1979).

The idea of nurses setting goals *for* patients and *with* patients and of implementing a plan to help individuals achieve goals is not a new one (Little and Carnevali, 1969; Nicholls, 1974). Nursing care plans have been used for many years to identify goals, methods to achieve them, and ways to evaluate whether or not goals have been achieved (Pardee, 1971; Nicholls and Wessells, 1977). If goals are achieved, a measure of effectiveness of care indicates quality assurance.

To date the movement in quality assurance has shown some agreement that evaluation of nursing must include process and outcomes. The excellent thinking, planning, and publishing of approaches and forms for initiating quality assurance programs in nursing have been used to suggest the construction of a Goal-Oriented Nursing Record that would extend and complement the Problem-Oriented Medical Record, and both would be used as a single patient record.* If nurses use a Goal-Oriented Nursing Record, they will document both process and outcomes in nursing situations because they will record the goals, the means to achieve them, and the process used to attain goals.

## Goal-Oriented Nursing Record

For many years nurses have discussed, published, and used a variety of forms to record nursing care plans (NCNA, 1974). A systematic record of the process of implementing a nursing care plan and the outcomes achieved should be part of the permanent record of the clients.

The passage of the law that established the Professional Standards

---

*To be known as POMR and GONR.

Review Organization has brought into focus the need for health care providers to develop professional standards that can measure the effectiveness of care (Geoffrey, 1977).

A variety of forms have been constructed, published, and used by a majority of nurses that proposes a logical and efficient way of educating students in nursing. In addition, these various forms were used to provide a systematic record of nursing care in hospitals and community agencies. Ideas were used from these sources as well as from publications of nurses who have seen the value of systematic recording of nursing care, and have published their adaptation of the problem-oriented medical record for use in nursing (Bonkowsky, 1972; Schell and Campbell, 1972; Aradine and Guthneck, 1974). Many of the ideas can be seen in the initial effort to develop a Goal-Oriented Nursing Record. This idea is different in that a dimension called *Goal List* is added since it places emphasis on the use of a theory of goal attainment described in this book. In addition, if nurses placed emphasis on goals to be attained in the nursing situation, they would approach a nursing situation with theoretical knowledge that helps to verify perceptions and the accuracy of the data gathered to identify problems and set goals.

## CHARACTERISTICS OF THE GOAL-ORIENTED NURSING RECORD

The Goal-Oriented Nursing Record (GONR) consists of five major elements: a data base, a problem list, a goal list, a plan, and progress notes.

The *data base* is composed of all information gathered about a person on entry into the health care system. This information includes the nursing history and health assessment; the physician history and physical examination; results of laboratory tests and x-ray examinations; and other sources, such as the family and social workers. In some health-care agencies nurses classify patients according to severity of illness or nursing care needs. In others, a systematic assessment of activities of daily living is made to determine the person's state of dependency and the need for assistance with nutrition, elimination, or mobility. One form, shown in Figure 6.1, can be used to record the data base. All professionals contribute to the information recorded.

From analysis of the data base, problems are identified, numbered, titled, and listed on the client's record. A problem list may or may not be a diagnosis. The *problem list,* shown in Figure 6.2, is updated as new information is gathered and interpreted and new problems identified and old ones resolved.

```
                        PATIENT DATA BASE
   NAME:_____ TIME:_____
   DATE:_____
   Admitted:
       Ambulatory___     Age_____     Assistive Devices     Informants
       Wheel chair___    Sex_____     Glasses_____       Patient___
       Stretcher_____    Weight___    Contact lens___       Family___
       Carried by___     Height___    Hearing aid___        Friend___
                                      Dentures_____       Other___
                                      Artificial
                                        eye_____
                                      Artificial
                                        limb_____
   Vital Signs:
     Blood pressure
         R arm____ Supine____ Sitting____ Standing____
         L arm____ Supine____ Sitting____ Standing____
     Temperature
         Oral____ Rectal____ Axillary____ Not taken____
     Pulse
         Apical____ Radial____ Other____ Not taken____
         Regular____ Slow____ Rapid____
         Irregular____ Weak____ Barely perceptible____
     Respirations
         Rate____ Regular____ Rapid____
         Shallow____ Ceased____ Cheyne-Stokes____
         Deep____ Labored____
   Chief complaint_____
   Duration of this Illness:
     Hours____ Weeks____ Years____ Days____ Months____
```

**Figure 6.1**  Data base form.

Previous Hospitalization:

Other Illnesses:

Experience with Hospitalization:

    Met expectations_____ Did not meet expectations_____

Effect of This Hospitalization:

    Creates problems_____ Financial_____ Employment_____ Child Care_____

    Insurance_____

Personal Habits:

    Skin:  Clean_____        Decubiti:        Bathing:

            Bruises_____    Location_____   By self_____

            Blisters_____     Odor_____       With assistance_____

            Lesions_____     Drainage_____   Prefers tub bath_____

            Rashes_____     None_____      Prefers shower_____

            Scars_____                               Other_____

            Wounds_____

    Mouth:

        Dentures: Upper_____ Lower_____ Partial upper_____ Partial lower_____

            Brushes teeth_____ Does not brush teeth_____

    Eating Habits:

        Usually eats 3 meals/day_____

        Usually omits breakfast_____ lunch_____ dinner_____

        Snacks regularly_____ No snacks_____

Food allergies_____

Food likes_____ Food dislikes_____

Special diet_____

**Figure 6.1** (Continued)

Personal Habits:

  Sleep/rest

    Usually arises at\_\_\_\_ Usually retires at\_\_\_\_

    Aides for sleep: None\_\_\_\_ Medication\_\_\_\_ (list)

    Difficulty sleeping\_\_\_\_

  Smoking

    Cigarettes\_\_\_\_ Number/day\_\_\_\_

    Cigars\_\_\_\_ Number/day\_\_\_\_

    Pipe\_\_\_\_

    Other\_\_\_\_ Has smoked in past\_\_\_\_

Exercise

  Type of exercise_____

  Frequency: Daily\_\_\_\_ Weekly\_\_\_\_ Severl times week\_\_\_\_ None\_\_\_\_

Elimination

  Bowels: Diarrhea\_\_\_\_ Constipation\_\_\_\_ Hemorrhoids\_\_\_\_

          Rectal pain\_\_\_\_ Uses laxatives\_\_\_\_

          Frequent enemas\_\_\_\_

          Regular\_\_\_\_ Frequency: daily\_\_\_\_ q other day\_\_\_\_

  Bladder: Frequency\_\_\_\_ Nocturia\_\_\_\_ Dysuria\_\_\_\_ Incontinence\_\_\_\_

           Pain/burning\_\_\_\_ Other\_\_\_\_

Social History:

  Habits: Smoking\_\_\_\_ Alcohol\_\_\_\_ Drugs.\_\_\_\_ Eating\_\_\_\_

  Marital status:_____

  Children_____

  Occupation:_____

  Education:_____

  Home situation\_\_\_\_ lives alone\_\_\_\_

                      lives with family\_\_\_\_

                      lives with friend\_\_\_\_

**Figure 6.1** (Continued)

Recreation:

    Hobbies:

        Active participant_____

Functional Review of Health:

    Neurologic_____

    Respiratory _____

    Circulatory_____

    Gastrointestinal_____

    Genitourinary_____

    Musculoskeletal_____

    Psychological Status_____

Current Medications (include dosage, etc.):

General Attitude:

Immediate Nursing Care:

**Figure 6.1** (Continued)

---

NAME: Mrs. Doe
DATE: 6-30-80          INITIAL PROBLEM LIST

Problem 1  Inability to move right arm and leg
Problem 2  Inability to speak sentences, but uses single words
Problem 3  Inability to feed self due to righthandedness
Problem 4  Inability to chew food on right side of mouth
Problem 5  Blood pressure elevated for this patient 190/110

**Figure 6.2** Problem list form for a sixty-year-old adult admitted to the hospital with a medical diagnosis of cerebral vascular accident.

The purposes of a problem list are numerous. A problem list is a guide for continuous assessment of subjective and objective signs and symptoms of a disturbance or interference in client's ability to function in usual roles. It is a guide to identify a nursing diagnosis and to plan for the patient's immediate nursing care. An overall advantage of a problem list is the consistent approach used by many nurses to implement a plan of nursing care. The list of nursing problems demonstrates an approach for coordination of nursing problems with medical and allied professionals' problems lists. The problem list documents the problems identified and those resolved by nursing care. Problems provide a way to identify some of the goals to be achieved in nursing situations.

A goal list is the third element in this nursing record. Examples of a goal list are shown in Figure 6.3. The purposes of a goal list are numer-

---

NAME: Mrs. Doe
DATE: 6-30-80             INITIAL GOAL LIST

Problem 1.  Inability to move right arm and leg
  Goal 1.   Observe and record patient status
  Process:  a. passive ROM exercises; coordinate with physical therapy
            b. neuro signs q 1 hour and report changes
            c. B/P q 1 hour and report changes
  Goal 2.   Provide comfort and safety
  Process:  a. position in bed and turn q 2 hours and support extremities especially right side
            b. skin care and protection of bony prominences
            c. mouth care
            d. call light within easy reach of left hand
            e. two people to move patient
  Goal 3.   Discuss nursing care and explain treatments; offer information so patient can participate in care
Problem 2.  Inability to speak sentences
  Goal 1.   Request referral to speech therapy
  Goal 2.   Speak slowly and in simple sentences; allow adequate time for responses; look in on patient frequently
  Goal 3.   Explain difficulty in speech to patient
Problem 3.  Inability to feed self
  Goal 1.   Feed patient; ask patient what food she prefers to eat first
  Goal 2.   Have patient try to use left hand to feed self; begin by holding piece of bread

Figure 6.3   Goal list form.

ous. Goals serve to guide nurses in the monitoring of the disturbances or interferences in patients and to be alert for any new patient information. Goals provide a means for nurse and clients to interact, to share information, to set mutual goals, to explore means and agree on means to achieve goals. A goal list provides for continuity of care. It focuses on clients' participation in decisions about their care. Interacting to set goals provides a way for growth and learning for both nurse and client. An overall advantage of a goal list in the client's record is that it provides a consistent and systematic approach to help individuals move toward a healthy state. This approach demonstrates individualized nursing care. This type of record facilitates nursing audits because it documents goals identified, a process for achieving them, and the outcomes of goals attained. Nursing audits are one part of quality assurance programs.

The fourth major element in the nursing record is a plan that is based on the assessment of the problem. A format borrowed from the Weed POMR is called SOAP. This format helps to describe and evaluate the problems (Weed, 1969).

- S = subjective data. How does the client perceive the problem? How does he/she feel about it?
- O = objective data. Examples are the physical examination, laboratory, and x-ray findings, objective measures that include activities of daily living and physiological parameters measured by blood pressure, pulse, and respiratory rate, and body temperature.
- A = assessment of the problem. From the data base, the problem is not only identified, but changes, positive or negative, are monitored, and action taken when necessary.
- P = plan. This includes the nursing diagnosis and the means agreed upon to resolve the problem and attain the goals. Client education may be an integral part of such a plan.

Relevant information in nursing situations is recorded in progress notes.

The fifth element in a Goal-Oriented Nursing Record is the use of *progress notes*. Weed (1969) identifies three types of progress notes: narrative, flow sheets, and final summary or discharge notes. Nurses record a concise summary of the progress of the client, and this is called a narrative note, as shown in Figure 6.4. For some populations of clients, flow sheets are used, as shown in Figure 6.5. They are designed and used for routine information or for continuous or repetitive recording of specific

```
NAME: Mrs. Doe
DATE: 6-30-80           PROGRESS NOTES – NARRATIVE

              Problem 1.  Observe and record patient status
10 A.M.       Goal 1.  S  complains of pain in back of head
                       O  holding head – facial muscles tense
                       A  appears in pain
                       P  check vital and neuro signs; stay with patient a
                          few minutes and check frequently
1 P.M.        Problem 1.  Observe and record patient status
              Goal 1.  S  no complaints of pain in head
                       O  neuro and vital signs stable
                       A  resting in bed
                       P  check neuro and vital signs q 3 hrs.
5 P.M.        Problem 3.  Inability to feed self
              Goal 1.  Feed patient
                       S  complains of numbness in right hand
                       O  cannot hold spoon or cup
                       A  needs continued help with feeding
                       P  help patient use left hand to feed self
```

**Figure 6.4** Progress notes—narrative form.

information, and for daily routine care. For example, if a patient in a hospital is being observed for neurological changes, nurses could use a reliable neurological nursing assessment tool as a flow sheet (Bolin, 1977). In addition, flow sheets may be used to show cumulative data, such as blood levels and special exercises at specified intervals. If information on flow sheets indicate changes in the client, progress notes are written in narrative form. A third type of progress note is the final summary or discharge note, shown in Figure 6.6. Each problem is discussed, each goal is stated, and information is written about whether or not the goal was attained. Any future goals are also written.

If nurses used a Goal-Oriented Nursing Record, a nursing audit would be facilitated in that the final summary would show problems identified and resolved and goals identified and attained. This type of record could be incorporated into any information system in any health care setting. This approach to nursing will help nurses increase their skills in making nursing diagnoses, in verifying accuracy in perceptions, in purposeful nurse–client interactions, and in helping individuals participate in making decisions that influence their life and their health.

NAME:
DATE:

PROGRESS NOTES – FLOW SHEET FORM
NEURO CHECK

| PUPILS | SIZE | STIMULUS – RESPONSE (S-R) | | MOTOR | |
|---|---|---|---|---|---|
| Reacts briskly  – 2 | = equal | Responds to commands | – 5 | Full spontaneous use | – 2 |
| Reacts slowly  – 1 | < less | Responds to name | – 4 | Moves to stimulus only | – 1 |
| No reaction  – 0 | > greater | Responds to shaking | – 3 | No movement | – 0 |
| | | Responds to pin prick | – 2 | | |
| LEVEL OF CONSCIOUSNESS (LOC) | | Responds to deep pain | – 1 | Right Upper extremity – RUE | |
| Alert & Oriented 3 | – 5 | No response | – 0 | Right lower extremity – RLE | |
| Alert & partially oriented | – 4 | | | Left upper extremity – LUE | |
| Lethargic but oriented | – 3 | TYPE OF RESPONSE (T.R.) | | Left lower extremity – LLE | |
| Lethargic & disoriented | – 2 | Complex Withdrawal | – 3 | | |
| Restless and/or combative | | Simple Withdrawal | – 2 | | |
| (confused) | – 2 | Postures | – 1 | | |
| Responds to stimulation | – 1 | Flaccid | – 0 | | |
| Unresponsive | 0 | | | | |

**Figure 6.5** Progress notes—flow sheet form. (Continued on pages 174–175.)

This neurological checklist is being kept on a young girl who was in an automobile accident two weeks previously. She sustained head, chest, and abdominal trauma. The injuries were repaired. The patient is comatose, responding only to such stimulation as that indicated on the form.

Copyright © 1977, American Journal of Nursing Company. Reproduced with permission from the *American Journal of Nursing*, vol. 77, no. 9, September 1977, p. 1479.

| TIME & DATE | PUPILS |  |  | L.O.C. | S-R | T.R. | MOTOR |  |  |  | TOTAL MAX. 25 |  |
|---|---|---|---|---|---|---|---|---|---|---|---|---|
|  | R | > = < | L |  |  |  | RUE | RLE | LUE | LLE |  |  |
|  |  |  |  |  |  |  |  |  |  |  |  |  |
|  |  |  |  |  |  |  |  |  |  |  |  |  |
|  |  |  |  |  |  |  |  |  |  |  |  | N |
|  |  |  |  |  |  |  |  |  |  |  |  | E |
|  |  |  |  |  |  |  |  |  |  |  |  | U |
|  |  |  |  |  |  |  |  |  |  |  |  | R |
|  |  |  |  |  |  |  |  |  |  |  |  | O |
|  |  |  |  |  |  |  |  |  |  |  |  | L |
|  |  |  |  |  |  |  |  |  |  |  |  | O |
|  |  |  |  |  |  |  |  |  |  |  |  | G |
|  |  |  |  |  |  |  |  |  |  |  |  | I |
|  |  |  |  |  |  |  |  |  |  |  |  | C |
|  |  |  |  |  |  |  |  |  |  |  |  | A |
|  |  |  |  |  |  |  |  |  |  |  |  | L |

**Figure 6.5** (Continued)

### Definitions

**Pupils:**
Self explanatory

**LOC:**
- (5) Alert & oriented × 3 = Awakens easily; oriented to person, place, time
- (4) Alert & partially oriented = Awakens easily but oriented in only 1 or 2 spheres
- (3) Lethargic but oriented = Slow to arouse, possibly slurred speech, but oriented × 3
- (2) Lethargic & disoriented = Slow to arouse, oriented in only 1 or 2 spheres or completely disoriented
- (2) Resless/combative (confused) = Spontaneously thrashing about in bed; striking out at others; inattentive to commands
- (1) Responds to stimulation only = exhibits only some type of withdrawal or posturing to stimulation
- (0) Unresponsive = No response of any kind

**S-R:**
- (5) Commands = appropriate response to orientation questions, compliance with hand grasp, toe wiggling, ec.
- (4) Name = Opens eyes to name, or gives some indication that he hears you (nods, moves, etc.) but does not follow all commands
- (3) Shaking = Responds only to vigorous physical stimulation
- (2) Pin prick = Responds to light pain applied with pin to trunk or extremities to elicit either withdrawal or posturing
- (1) Deep pain = Responds only to mandibular pressure, periorbital rub, sternal rub, or pinch
- (0) No response = Nothing elicited by any stimulus

**T-R:**
- (3) Complex withdrawal = withdrawal & attempt to remove stimulus
- (2) Simple withdrawal = only withdrawal from stimulus
- (1) Posturing = decorticate — head, arms & hand flexed
  decerebrate — head extended, arms extended & pronated, back arched
- (0) Flaccid = No response

**Motor:**
- (2) Spontaneous use = Moves designated extremity or extremities with or without any stimulation
- (1) To stimulus only = Response only to touch, pin, or deep pain
- (0) No movement = Nothing

Weakness of any extremity is indicated by writing "weaker" under the appropriate column.

**Figure 6.5** (Continued)

---

NAME:
DATE: 7-14-80     PROGRESS NOTES — FINAL SUMMARY

Problem 1. Able to move right arm; leg needs support for movement
  Goal 1. Partially attained — able to move right arm and use hand with caution
  Goal 2. Attained — skin intact
Problem 2. Inability to speak sentences
  Goal 1. Attained — speech therapy involved in Rx
  Goal 2. Attained — patient able to speak simple sentences
  Goal 3. Attained — patient thanked nurses for their explanations of events and their patience in assisting with feeding and speech
Problem 3. Inability to feed self
  Goal 1. Patient able to use left hand to feed self; right hand movement permits use of right hand to feed self

Summary: Patient partially recovered and can help self in daily hygiene. Needs leg brace, walker, and assistance in walking. To continue physical therapy after discharge and to be seen by nurse practitioner and speech therapist.

---

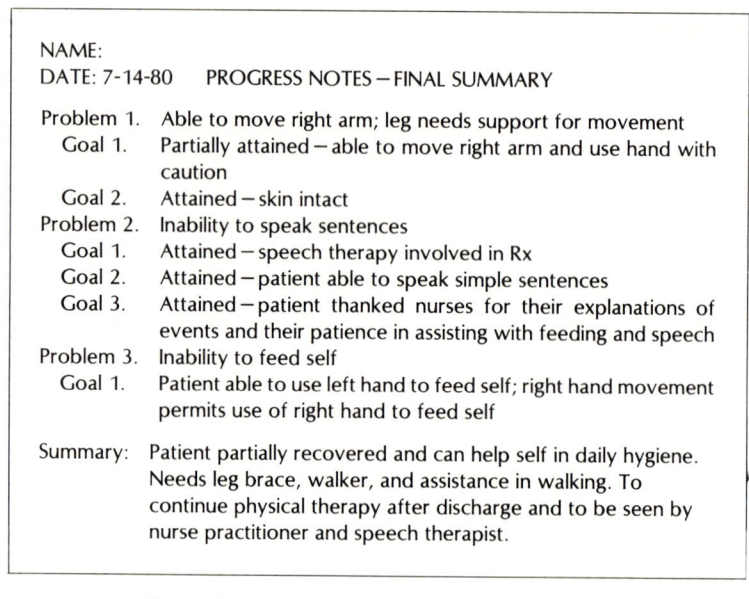

**Figure 6.6** Progress notes—final summary form.

**Theory, nursing process, record system.** A theory of goal attainment provides a theoretical basis for nursing process as it demonstrates a way for nurses to interact purposefully with clients. In the course of those interactions, information is shared, mutual goals are set, and clients are asked to participate in decisions about the means to achieve goals. A plan is implemented. There is continuous assessment and evaluation through the nurse–client interactions, nurse observations, and measurement of physiological variables.

Medical diagnosis and treatment are well known in the health field. Nursing diagnosis as a basis for planning nursing care has been discussed for 20 years but only recently has the term been given explicit emphasis by nurses (Gebbie and Lavin, 1975; Gordon, 1976).

The fourth National Conference on the Classification of Nursing Diagnosis was held in April 1980. The participants discussed the possibility of a conceptual framework that would organize the nomenclature into a system. The concepts of the goal-attainment theory presented in this book offer one way to organize diagnostic categories that deal with personal and interpersonal systems.

## Summary

A theory of goal attainment provides basic knowledge of nursing as a process of interactions that leads to transactions in nursing situations. A Goal-Oriented Nursing Record facilitates the use of this theory in nursing education and nursing practice. In addition, the Goal-Oriented Nursing Record provides a systematic approach to making nursing diagnosis from the client data base, especially the data collected by nurses' observations and measurements. The nursing diagnosis identifies the disturbances, problems, or concerns about which patients seek help. These problems make up the problem list. From this list nurses develop a goal list and identify immediate and future goals for each client. The progress notes in the record show the process used to achieve goals. Outcomes are identified as goals attained. Goals attained are measures of effectiveness of nursing care. This approach provides a built-in quality assurance system. The Goal-Oriented Nursing Record used in conjunction with a Problem-Oriented Medical Record can provide a structure for professional collaboration and cooperation. The effectiveness of health care can be evaluated.

## Bibliography

Aradine, C. R., and Guthneck, M., The Problem Oriented Record in a Family Health Service, *American Journal of Nursing*, 74, July 1974, 1108-1112.

Beeker, B. A., and Kinball, L. S., Evaluation of Goal Achievement in the Care of an Adolescent with a Traumatic Injury, in *Nursing Standards and Nursing Process*, edited by M. E. Nicholls and V. G. Wessells, Contemporary Publishing, Wakefield, Massachusetts, 1977, 135-139.

Bircher, A., On the Development and Classification of Diagnosis, *Nursing Forum*, 14, 1975, 10-29.

Bjorn, J. C., and Cross, H. D., *Problem Oriented Private Practice of Medicine: System for Comprehensive Health Care*, Modern Hospital Press, McGraw-Hill, Chicago, 1970, p. 67.

Blount, M., Green, S. S., Hamory, A.. Kinney, A. B., and C. W. Sanborn, Documenting with the Problem-Oriented Record Systems, *American Journal of Nursing*, 78, September 1978, 1539-1542.

Bolin, K., Assessing the Status of Neurological Patients, *American Journal of Nursing*, 77(9), September 1977, 1478-1479.

Bonkowsky, M. L., Problem Oriented Medical Records: Adapting the POMR to Community Child Health Care, *Nursing Outlook*, 20(8), August 1972, 517.

Gebbie, K. M., and Lavin, M. A., *Classification of Nursing Diagnosis,* Mosby, St. Louis, 1975.

Geoffrey, L. S., Professional Standards Review Organizations (PSROs), in *Nursing Standards and Nursing Process,* edited by M. E. Nicholls and V. G., Wessels, Contemporary Publishing, Wakefield, Massachusetts, 1977, pp. 27-30.

Given, B., Given, C. W., Simmons, S., and Lewis, E., Relationships of Processes of Care to Patient Outcomes, *Nursing Research,* 28(2) March-April 1979, 85-93.

Gordon, M., Nursing Diagnosis and the Diagnostic Process, *American Journal of Nursing,* 76(8), August 1976, 1298-1300.

Hofing, A. L., McGugin, M. B., and Merkel, S. I., The Importance of Maintenance in Implementing Change: An Experience with Problem-Oriented Recording, *The Journal of Nursing Administration,* 9, December 1979, 43-48.

Hurst, J. W., and Waker, H. K. (eds.), *The Problem-Oriented System,* MedCom Press, New York, 1972.

Kane, D., The Computer in Nursing, in *The Problem Oriented System,* edited by J. W. Hurst and H. K. Waker, MedCom Press, New York, 1972, pp. 251-257.

Little, D., and Carnevali, D., *Nursing Care Planning,* Lippincott, Philadelphia, 1978.

Mayers, M. G., Norby, R. B., and Watson, A. B., *Quality Assurance for Patient Care: Nursing Perspective,* Appleton-Century-Crofts, New York, 1977.

Mundinger, M., and Janson, G., Developing a Nursing Diagnosis, *Nursing Outlook,* 23(2), February 1975, 94-98.

Nicholls, M. E., Quality Control in Patient Care, *American Journal of Nursing,* 74(3), March 1974, p. 456-459.

Nicholls, M. E., Terminology in Quality Assurance, in *Nursing Standards and Nursing Process,* edited by M. E. Nicholls and V. G. Wessells, Contemporary Publishing, Wakefield, Massachusetts, 1977, 31-38.

*Nursing Clinics of North America,* Symposium on Problem-Oriented Record and Symposium on Quality Assurance, 9(2), Saunders, Philadelphia, June 1974.

Pardee, G., et al., Patient Care Evaluation Is Every Nurses' Job, *American Journal of Nursing,* 71(10), October 1971, 1958-1960.

Schell, P. L., and Campbell, A. T., POMR—Not Just Another Way to Chart, *Nursing Outlook,* 25(8), August 1972, 510-514.

Weed, L. L., *Medical Records, Medical Education, and Patient Care,* Case Western Reserve University Press, Cleveland, 1969.

Wessells, V. G., Nursing Process and Quality Control, in *Nursing Standards and Nursing Process,* edited by M. E. Nicholls and V. G. Wessells, Contemporary Publishing, Wakefield, Massachusetts, 1977.

Woody, M., and Mallison, M., The Problem-Oriented System of Patient-Centered Care, *American Journal of Nursing,* 73(7), July 1973, 1168-1175.

# Index

Activities of daily living, 1
Actions, human, 59-60, 102
Acts, human, 59-60, 102
Age, 114, 148
Authority, characteristics of, 123
  concept of, 122
  definition of, 124
  implications for nursing, 124-125

Body image, characteristics of, 32
  concept of, 31-34
  definition of, 32-33
  implications for nursing, 33-34

Communication, characteristics of, 69-74
  concept of, 62-63
  definition of, 69, 146
  diagrams, 63, 65-66
  implications for nursing, 75-79
  information, 80-81
  interpersonal, 67-69
  intrapersonal, 67
  models, 63-66
  nonverbal, 71-73
  principles, 68
  process, 69, 74
  touch, 71-72, 77-78
  verbal, 69-70
Concepts:
  authority, 122
  body image, 31-34
  communication, 62-63
  decision making, 130-131
  growth and development, 29-31, 142
  health, 4-8
  interactions, 59-62, 84-85, 144
  organization, 116-117
  perception, 20-21, 61, 80, 88
  power, 126-127
  role, 89-91
  self, 26-29
  space, 34-40
  status, 129-130
  stress, 95-97
  time, 40-46
  transactions, 80-81

179

use of, 13
Conceptual framework, 10-13, 141

Decision making, characteristics of, 132
  concept of, 130-131
  definition of, 132-133
  implications for nursing, 133-134
Diagrams:
  classification system of nurse/patient interaction, 156
  communication, 63, 65-66
  dynamic interacting systems, 11
  goal attainment, theory of, 157
  human interaction process, 61, 145

Environment, 1, 5-6, 66, 69, 141

Family, 1, 113-114

Goal attainment, 1, 141, 163, 176
Goal oriented nursing record, characteristics of, 133-134 164-165
  database, 166-169
  goal list, 171
  plan, 171
  problem list, 170
  progress notes, 172-176
Goals, 3-8, 13, 145, 163-164, 170
Goal setting, mutual, 142, 151
Groups, 10-11, 113
Growth and development, characteristics of, 30-31
  concept of, 29-31, 142
  definition of, 148

Health, characteristics of, 5-6
  concept of, 4-8

definition of, 5
implications for nursing, 7-8
indicators, 5-7
promotion, 6-7

Illness, 5, 163, 165, 169-170
Individuals, 19-20, 47, 62, 141, 143
Information, 62-66, 133-134
Interactions, assumptions, 143-144
  characteristics, 62, 80-84
  concept of, 59-62, 84-85, 144
  definition of, 85, 145
  diagrams, 61, 145
  implications for nursing, 83-87
  information, 62
  process of, 60-61, 143-145, 152, 177
Interpersonal Systems, 10, 59, 83, 88, 142-144

Medical record, problem oriented, 133, 163-164

Nurses, characteristics of, 2
  code of, 12
  functions, 1, 8-9
Nursing, definition of, 144
  diagnosis, 172, 176-177
  domain, 1, 2
  effectiveness of care, 8, 142, 164, 177
  goals, 3, 13
  propositions, 149
  situation, 2, 88, 102
  theory, 141-149, 156-157
  values, 12, 13

Organization, characteristics of, 116-118

their orientation and had knowledge of the hospital and the patient care unit. The variable of working in a strange environment can limit the time and kind of interactions between nurses and patients. Following an explanation of the study, those nurses who volunteered signed an informed consent form.

The patients who were assigned to the nurses who volunteered were then contacted by the investigator, the study was explained to each patient, and those who volunteered also signed an informed consent form. The observation period was planned from 9–11 A.M. since this was the time when multiple interactions were taking place. The sample consisted of 17 cases.

The verbal and nonverbal behaviors of nurses and patients were recorded as raw data. Data analysis was facilitated by using the operational definition of transactions inductively developed prior to conducting the study. The behaviors in the operational definition were assigned numbers one through seven for coding purposes.

## RESULTS

The frequencies and percentages of the six categories in the interactions are shown in Table 5.1. Goals were attained in 12 of the 17 cases studied, or 70 percent of the sample.

Three questions were asked. First, what elements in nurse–patient interactions lead to transactions? Elements identified in nurse–patient interactions that lead to transactions were the identification of a problem, concern, or disturbance in the patient environment. Nurse and patient explored the situation, shared information, and mutually set goals. They explored means to resolve the problem and achieve the goal, and both moved forward to implement a plan and attain a goal.

The second question was: what are the relationships between the elements in the interactions that lead to transactions? The interactions were characterized by verbal and nonverbal communication between nurse and patient. The first six behaviors in the operational definition were coded as distinct elements in the interaction. These behaviors were called *predictor variables* or *independent variables*. If these behaviors were present in the data, the possibility that transactions would take place and goals would be achieved could be predicted. The seventh element in the definition was called a *criterion* or *dependent variable* because if transactions occurred, goals were attained and outcomes could be measured. Transactions may therefore be considered a measure of effectiveness of nursing care.

tions. Transactions are defined as goals achieved through mutual goal setting and implementing the means to achieve goals. Goals are expected outcomes in each nursing situation. Previous studies in perception, interaction, interpersonal relations, and nursing process have investigated one part of an interaction between two person's verbal or nonverbal behaviors. Some studies reported the content of the interaction and some the duration of the interaction. Except for studies such as Orlando's (1972), few have reported verbal and nonverbal behaviors in natural situations. One major difference in this study and all others is that it described the nurse–patient interaction process that leads to goal attainment.

## METHOD

A nonparticipant observation technique was used systematically to collect data about nurse–patient interactions in natural settings. The setting was a large medical center in a metropolitan area in a general medical and a general surgical patient care unit.

## PROCEDURE

Four graduate students were trained in the nonparticipant observation technique during a one-week training period. Several hours were spent in a quiet conference room viewing a movie in which nurse–patient interactions were observed and recorded. Ten-minute segments of the movie were shown; the observers recorded verbal and nonverbal behaviors on the form used in the study. Observers were paired; while one observed verbal behaviors, the other observed nonverbal behaviors. The recorded observations were analyzed, and a reliability of .90 was achieved. Two 10-minute time periods were used for observations in a patient care unit that was not used in the study. These recorded observations were analyzed, and a reliability of .90 was achieved.

## SAMPLE

The study was approved by the Institutional Review Board of the hospital for the protection of rights of human subjects prior to asking nurses and patients to volunteer to be observed. One informed consent form was used for nurses and a second form used for patients. The nurses had to be employed full-time by the hospital for at least 6 months and in that particular setting for 3 months to ensure that the nurses had completed

INDEX • 181

analysis of, 116
concept of, 116-117
definition of, 119
formal-informal, 117, 120
implications for nursing,
 119-121
Outcomes, 1, 142-143

Perception, application to
 nursing, 24-25, 141-142
characteristics of, 22-23, 81
concept of, 20-21, 61, 80, 88
definition of, 24, 146
Personal systems, 19-20
Philosophical assumptions, 143-144
Power, characteristics of, 126-127
concept of, 126-127
definition of, 127
implications for nursing,
 128-129
Process, 2, 9, 24, 31, 42-45,
 60-61, 79, 86, 144, 157
Propositions, 149

Role, application to nursing, 94-95
characteristics of, 91-92
concepts of, 89-91
definition of, 93, 147

Self, characteristics of, 26-27
concept of, 26-29
definition of, 27-28
implications for nursing,
 29, 142
Space, application to nursing,
 38-40
characteristics of, 36-37
concept of, 34-40
definition of, 37-38, 148
Status, characteristics of, 129
concept of, 129-130
definition of, 129-130
implications for nursing, 130

Stress, characteristics of, 97-98
concept of, 95-97
definition of, 98, 147
implications for nursing,
 99, 100-102
Systems:
communication systems, 63-67
dynamic interacting systems,
 11, 61, 141
interpersonal systems, 10-11, 59
personal systems, 10, 19
social systems, characteristics of,
 114
concept of, 11-12, 113
definition of, 115

Theory, application to nursing,
 133, 157-163, 176-177
characteristics of, 142-150, 156
concepts, definition of, 144-145
descriptive testing, 150-155
hypotheses, 156
operational definition, 150-151
philosophical assumptions, 143-144
propositions, 143-144, 149
schematic diagram, 157
Time, application to nursing, 45-46
characteristics of, 42-44
communication, 42
concept of, 40-46
definition of, 44-45, 148
perspectives, 41-42
Touch, 71-72, 77-78
Transactions, characteristics of,
 23, 82
concept of, 80-81
definition of, 1, 82, 147
implications for nursing, 82-83
operational definition, 150-151
study of values, 81, 88-89

Values, 12, 26, 81